WORK IN

THE ATHLETE'S PLAN
FOR REAL RECOVERY
AND WINNING RESULTS

ERIN TAYLOR

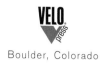

VELO PRESS

Boulder, Colorado

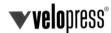

3002 Sterling Circle, Suite 100
Boulder, CO 80301–2338 USA

VeloPress is the leading publisher of books on endurance sports. Focused on cycling, triathlon, running, swimming, and nutrition/diet, VeloPress books help athletes achieve their goals of going faster and farther. Preview books and contact us at velopress.com.

Distributed in the United States and Canada by Ingram Publisher Services

A Cataloging-in-Publication record for this book is available from the Library of Congress.
ISBN 978-1-937715-77-9

This paper meets the requirements of ANSI/NISO Z39.48-1992 (Permanence of Paper).

Cover design by Kevin Roberson
Interior design by Kevin Roberson and Vicki Hopewell
Photos by Claire Pepper, except pp. viii and x by Jess Barnard and p. 189 by Sarah Robinson
Women's apparel provided by Oiselle

18 19 20 / 10 9 8 7 6 5 4 3 2 1

WORK IN

Heather
Elizabeth
Thomas
2019

To you, the athletes

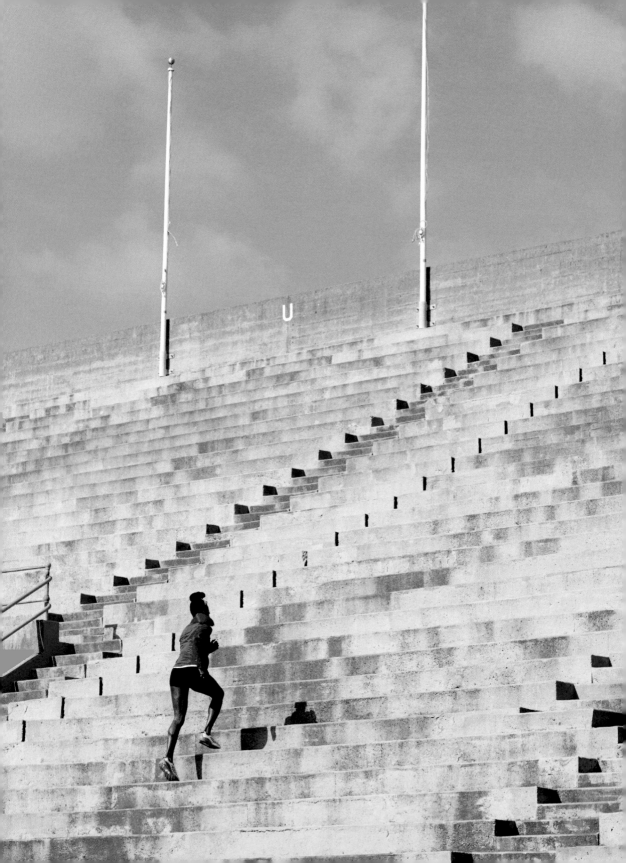

CONTENTS

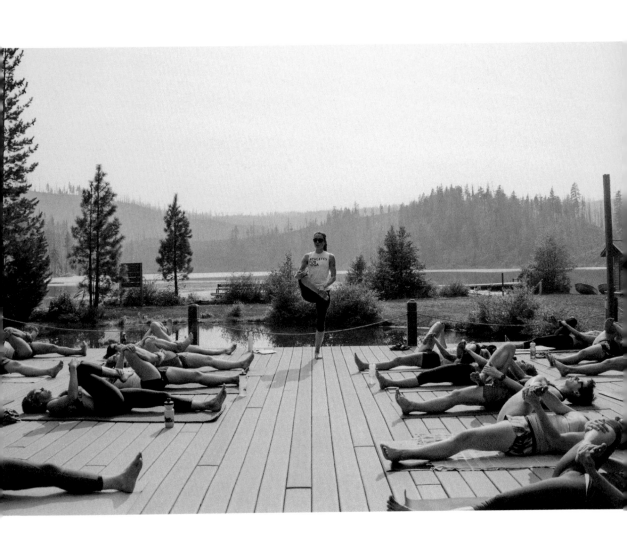

PREFACE

The first time I seriously explored meditation and yoga as a way to aid athletic recovery was at a weekend retreat with a yoga teacher known for her expertise in restorative yoga. The room was filled to capacity and the people there weren't messing around. The teacher began by acknowledging how difficult these practices are and the commitment required to access the benefits. She guided us to settle in and begin our first meditation. We hadn't gotten 10 seconds into the session when I farted—loud. I couldn't stop laughing. Even my husband—an incredibly good sport who was on a bolster next to me—shot me a sideways grin like, "What is wrong with you?"

As I continued to giggle, I finally became aware of a strong resistance to relaxation. It was limiting me. As a type A athlete, I had long found the concept foreign and counterproductive, and I was laughing out of discomfort because I was struggling to allow myself to recover in a meaningful way. This wasn't a choice; it was a habit. I couldn't switch gears mentally or physically even though I was at a restorative yoga workshop on purpose.

I tried anyway. And on the last day it paid off. After hours of sitting and daydreaming over the course of the weekend, acutely aware of the agitation of my stiff hips and strained back from my workouts earlier that week, I experienced a moment of absolute relaxed clarity like none I'd ever felt up to that point. As I sat, my mind and body were completely relaxed and at ease. I was overcome by a feeling of spaciousness—thoughts emptied from my head, and tension released from my body. It felt like I had "come home."

That moment forever changed the way I perceive the practice of mental focus and physical relaxation, and it has motivated me to continue. Over the years I have found that

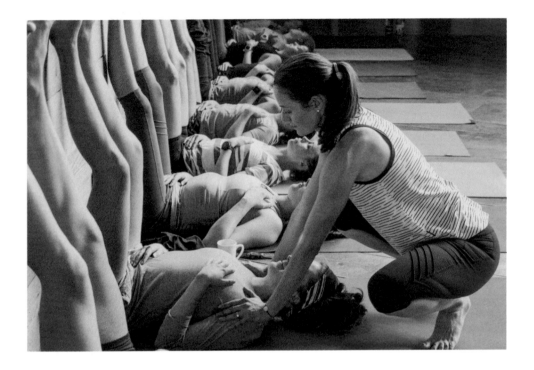

the more I practice, the more moments like this I experience, which not only continues to fuel my motivation to practice but also makes me more effective in everything I do.

Whether after work or after a workout, it feels good to come home after a long day or hard effort. For me, working in is the same thing. It helps me "come home" to myself—relax back into my body—so I can gain perspective, absorb my effort, and regather my strength for what lies ahead.

I hope that you too will feel at home in yourself every time you work in. And enjoy all of the wins that result.

WORK IN FOR THE WIN

Athletes are familiar with going hard—after all, working out gets results. What few are familiar with is resting easy—working in also gets results. When you go hard you have to rest hard, too.

We live in a world where every millisecond matters. As athletes we are goal oriented and highly invested in achievement—we do everything possible to gain competitive advantage and win. We're connected and aware, tracking pace and distance and all available physiological metrics related to performance. We leverage every aspect of preparation—from personal coaching to high-tech gadgets—in an effort to refine and optimize our output and bring our goals within reach. But even with all the knowledge gained and miles logged, most of us still aren't aware how much working in matters. We have all this data about our workout, and in some cases advice about when to stop, but it doesn't tell us what to do next, nor is it tracking our recovery—our work in. And for those looking to stretch the boundaries of their potential, it's working in that's the real game changer.

Most athletes know recovery is important. From cooldown routines to meditation apps to self-massage tools, the means to aid the process have gained consideration and adoption in recent years. This is a step in the right direction, but we still lack the practical understanding and skills to recover in a meaningful way. The misconception remains that working out is the only path to increased performance. As a result, recovery is one of the least planned, underutilized tools to optimize performance. It's falsely perceived as a given on "rest days" and a separate, less important endeavor that happens by default when we're not working out.

The reality is that, in sports and in life, recovery is as important and equally as productive as everything else that you do. You need relaxation after exertion. Not only

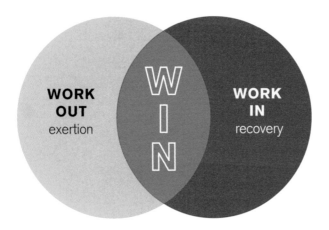

that, when used together in an integrated way, working out and working in will help you become more balanced and resilient and close the gap between where you are now and where you want to be. If you're serious about your goals, you should be asking:

⇒ How do I recognize when it's time to slow down and allow myself to stop?
⇒ And when I do stop, what should I do?

This book exists to help you answer these questions for yourself, and it is designed to elevate your athletic experience using a simple framework that will help you feel the difference—and step up from bronze to silver, and from silver to gold. Like working out, working in requires an intentional approach. Luckily, you can activate recovery when you need it most and make a real impact in as little as 5 minutes a day.

Use these tools to work in for the win:

TRY IT: Quick tips to help you recharge anytime, anywhere.

WORK IN: Do the routines to optimize your recovery—on purpose.

GET REAL: Become more intentional and effective in your approach by thinking about what you're doing, and why.

Embracing recovery will make you a better athlete. Your body is asking you to work in. It's time to listen and respond.

Ready, set, recover!

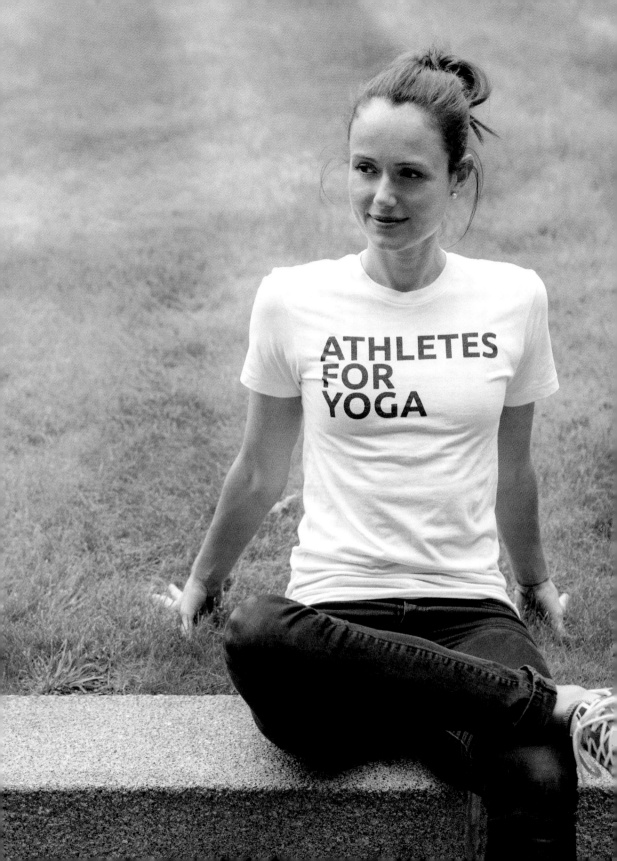

01

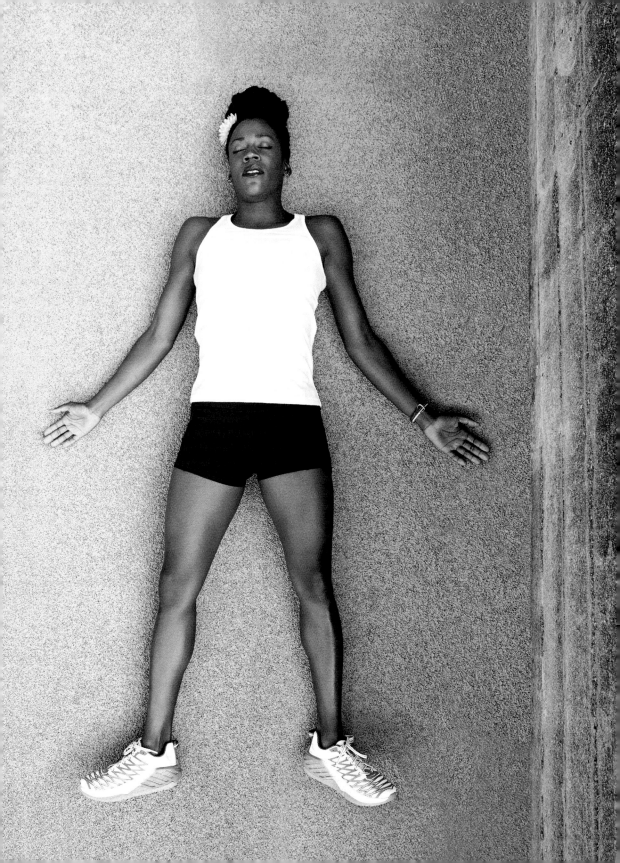

RETHINK RECOVERY

It's time to get real about recovery. You might already know that yoga and meditation can help athletic recovery, but the dots have to be connected. You have to do more than go to a yoga class, or close your eyes and set a timer. You'll get very little out of going through the motions of restorative activities—on or off the mat. To optimize recovery you have to reset your perception of rest and break your habit of resisting it.

It's how you work in that matters. It must become your new normal, a given every day. To do this, you have to bravely endeavor in the opposite direction of your usual mode of operation in order to blend your working out and working in to full advantage. The good news is that you already possess everything you need to recover for real right now. With practice, you can make the process of working in as habitual as working out. And it feels good, too.

REAL RECOVERY = Making recovery a practical,
integrated part of daily life

It's fitting that working out is called exactly that. It's an output, an energy expenditure in which you work against external factors—your feet hitting the pavement, your legs powering your bike, your arms pulling your body through the water, your muscles contracting against the weight in order to get the results you need to achieve your goals.

With practice, you've built your tolerance for working out. But without practicing your work in, you'll build more resistance than tolerance for real recovery.

Going hard comes easy because you are familiar with output. There's comfort in the familiarity of pushing yourself to your limits. You're conditioned to keep going and muscle your way through challenges. You attach a great deal of value to training, and rightfully so. And naturally, it feels counterintuitive that endeavoring in the opposite direction—working in—will move you toward your goals.

Sports and fitness pursuits are becoming more extreme, requiring more hours, more miles, and more output in general. Working out is not always a conscious choice you make; it's a familiar, comfortable—and often unintentional—habit. It's a hard habit to break, and one that makes you quick to say yes to doing more. You say yes enthusiastically because you're passionate about what you're doing and willing to do what

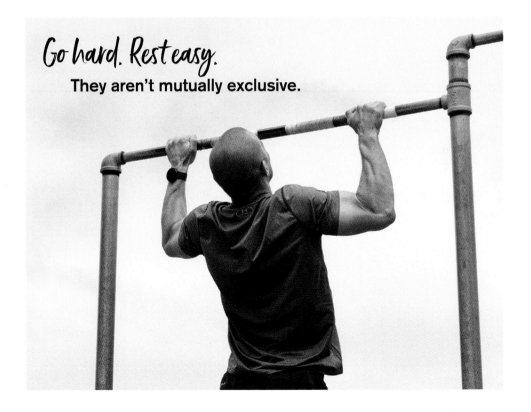

Go hard. Rest easy.
They aren't mutually exclusive.

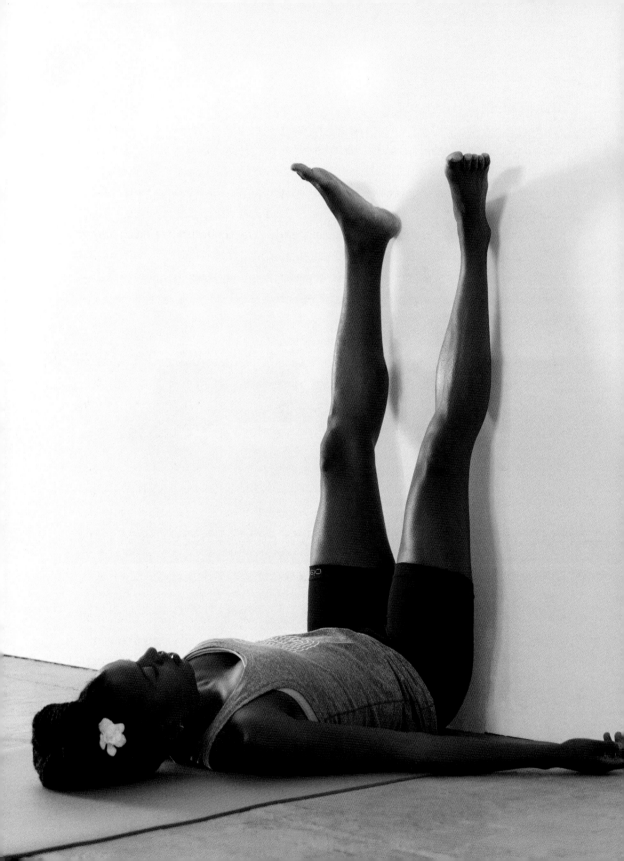

it takes to win. But do you recognize when the workload is too heavy? And if you do, can you say yes to recovery with the same level of conviction? Or do you agonize about skipping a training session? Saying yes to going hard is much easier than saying yes to resting easy because working out feels like progress and working in feels like a hard stop.

Athletes also fail to decelerate because they don't recognize just how much they're doing and how tired they are. When you are always going it becomes increasingly difficult to distinguish between work and rest, between energy and fatigue. Being amped up feels normal. Your body forgets that there are other, equally important gears and paces. But frazzled is not fit. And being injured sucks.

Mental and physical stress—from the aches and pains that often linger post-workout to the pressures of competition—can wreak havoc on even the strongest of athletes. Depriving your body of focused recovery during a particularly gruelling training program can cause your training to go haywire. Workouts tax your muscles, and those tissues cannot grow without ample time to repair. Energy is a limited yet renewable resource. It must be replenished through nutrition and rest. Without continual input, energy becomes more and more depleted, creating a deficit over time. The resulting fatigue lowers your mood and negatively affects your mental state, and, when left unaddressed, it can increase the risk of depression. All of these factors detract from the training you have put in and threaten your performance, leaving you feeling heavy and lethargic—and possibly even stagnant.

You know you can *power through*, but overpowering your body is *not winning*.

In pursuit of better performance, you keep looking for more ways to maximize output. But your body is already saturated with the physiological effects of your workouts. Many of these are not only positive but critical for growth: You become stronger as you train your body and mind to endure exertion, and chemicals like endorphins and serotonin linger post-workout, making you feel good—as does the satisfaction of a big effort or key training block completed. But continually muscling through can place an unsustainable load of stress on your system. While stress is a crucial ingredient for growth, systematically overdoing it puts you at risk of under-recovering, which is the root cause of overtraining.

UNDER-RECOVERING = Trading input for more output

Without ample daily rest you fall into a deficit as you become oversaturated with the stress of your training, soaking you in a 24/7 bath of cortisol and other stress hormones because your body still thinks it's fighting through even when your workout is over. Your tissues actually break down under overtraining conditions. When you're in a hot bath and your fingertips become wrinkled and puckered, you have to get out of the water so they become smooth again. It's the same with your muscles and your mind. Rest factors into building strength and endurance because it takes time to adapt to the forces involved. Without rest, not only is it impossible to progress in a meaningful way because your hard work can't pay off to its maximum, but it's more likely that you'll regress. Continuing to push is like being on a treadmill, running without advancing. Instead of looking for more ways to put out, consider input as a tool to maximize your output. Stepping off the treadmill halts the output so that you can absorb all your hard work and reap the rewards. It gives you the opportunity to actually feel what you've done. It's also powerful injury and burnout mitigation. You can and should keep going hard. But don't miss out on the other end of the spectrum and underachieve because you are under-recovering.

You've *built up your tolerance* for the discomfort of working out. Are you *brave enough* to build the same tolerance for the discomfort of *working in?*

Slow Down Significantly to Accelerate Radically

Working in—intentional, optimized recovery—is largely uncharted territory for athletes. It's like outer space—expansive and full of possibility and right in front of our eyes. To maximize your athletic potential, and to make the most of all your workouts, you have to shift your focus to the expanse within.

Don't mistake working in for "stopping" or lack of action—it will not happen by default when you're not actively training. Working out is an intentional expenditure, and so is working in. Just because recovery involves rest doesn't mean that it's a passive, sleepy state. Working in is a purposeful, engaged approach to optimizing your recovery.

Just like you have to fuel yourself with proper nutrition so that you have energy to feel and perform your best, you have to recover adequately every day so that your body and mind can return to equanimity and you can recharge for your next session.

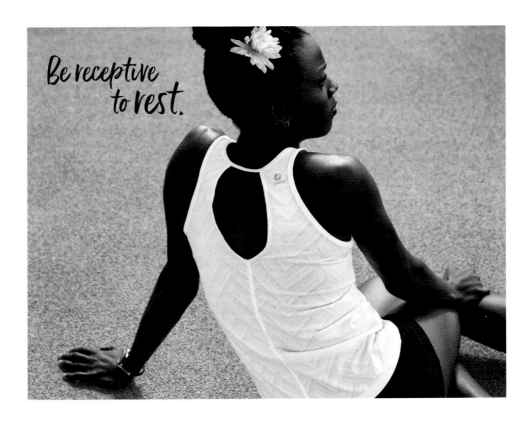

REST DAYS DON'T ENSURE RECOVERY

Dedicated rest days are important, but don't confuse them with recovery because they're not the same thing and the two don't necessarily go hand in hand. Recovery is what your body is designed to do after training—a return to neutral that keeps your systems balanced and optimized and advances you toward your goals. A rest day is a dedicated time for recovery, void of any training related activities. The problem is, too many athletes have lost the ability to transition from working to not working, making it impossible to effectively recover on rest days.

Most athletes—and humans in general—are so geared up that they struggle to wind down and recover even when the opportunity presents itself (like a rest day). As much as you might like the idea of relaxing and even value the importance of dedicated recovery time, if your habit is to do the opposite it can be tough to give yourself permission to slow down. And when you do finally create space to move in the opposite direction, it's likely to feel uncomfortable. You have to practice the transition. If a triathlete doesn't practice the transition from biking to running, the body is confused and it will show in the performance. Similarly, your body will resist rest if you don't intentionally practice the transition from training to recovering.

Scheduling rest days is admirable, but it's not enough. It's working in that helps your body become receptive to rest. You apply strength and courage to keep going even when your workouts get tough, and working in works the same way—don't back down. Working in helps you to manage the discomfort of shifting gears; it facilitates a smooth and effective transition from` work to rest so that you can assimilate all of your effort, truly rest on your rest days, and recover for real.

Effective recovery isn't a
guaranteed result of a rest day.

Consistent input is the counterbalance to your consistent output. It helps you maintain stronger awareness of where you're at by pulling you out of the oversaturation of output so that you can adjust your cadence based on what is actually happening.

Use Your Nervous System

We tend to approach recovery with different tools and techniques—foam rollers, compression, massage, physical therapy, and even different approaches to sleep and nutrition. It's ironic that our restorative activities tend to first focus on our muscles, even though they are the part of our body that naturally recovers the quickest because they receive direct blood flow. You might be less aware of the system that has the biggest impact on your ability to restore body and mind after a big output: your nervous system.

Your autonomic nervous system regulates your body's instinctive, unconscious actions and influences the function of your internal organs. It includes your brain, spinal cord, and nerves; and it regulates many bodily functions, such as heart rate, digestion, blood pressure, and respiration—all of which keep you going and moving forward, and play a critical role in movement, exertion, and ultimately performance.

Your nervous system sounds the alarm by way of a chemical stress response when you're confronted with life-threatening events, often referred to as the "fight or flight" response. This is governed by your sympathetic nervous system (SNS), which under duress triggers a reaction where blood pressure increases to supply more oxygen to your brain and muscles, and all your systems are optimized for you to defend yourself or run for your life. Your focus narrows to meet the challenge. This is all incredibly useful if you're attacked in a dark alley. Or running from a tiger. Or, more likely, when the fight is on for first place or a new PR in the last 100 meters of your race.

On the opposite end of the spectrum, your relaxation response is governed by your parasympathetic nervous system (PNS)—this is where you rest and digest. Since your nervous system is designed for self-preservation, your PNS should kick in once threatening events have passed to slow your heart rate, aid in digestion, and return you to a baseline of calm. It broadens your perspective and helps you to be more aware of where you're at so that you can more clearly discern the most appropriate course

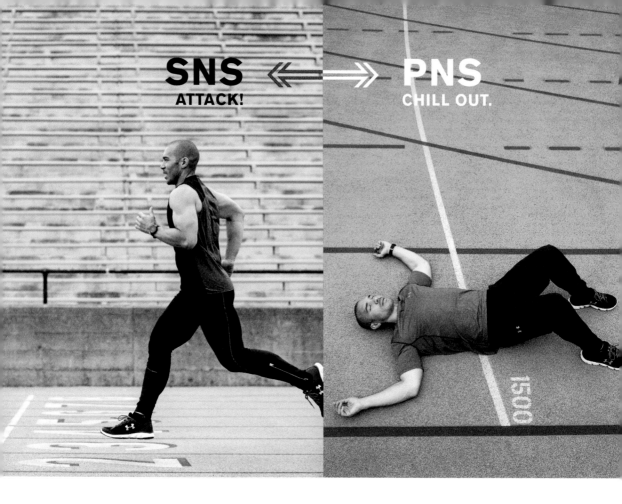

SNS
ATTACK!

PNS
CHILL OUT.

of action, rather than just react. Strengthening your PNS increases your resilience and helps you to more easefully manage whatever comes at you.

The problem is that because we are doing so much, all the time, we get stuck in fight or flight and can't wind down. As a result the SNS response is easily triggered by normal day-to-day occurrences like rushing to get to the gym, or triaging a full email inbox. When you're in this frame of mind your brain perceives the threat of failing to hit your pace in a key training session the same way it perceives the threat that you might be late for your meeting because you're stuck in traffic. While you need to get fired up to nail your workout, getting amped up in gridlock confuses your body with unnecessary stress and deprives you of spending time in a more relaxed state. The physiological design of the nervous system is disrupted by the pace of life. Stress management might be a big motivator of your workouts, but without consistent, effective PNS activation you're merely creating a vicious cycle of SNS stimulation.

HOW DO I KNOW WHEN TO STOP?

It's hard to know when it's okay to slow your roll and, more important, when to allow yourself to stop. Don't wait for someone else to tell you to rest. You don't need permission. You are the only one who can put your foot on the brakes. Your performance and overall well-being will suffer if you power on. You might feel too busy to slow down, but, ironically, it is the times when you're most frazzled that it's critical for you to work in.

Your body will tell you everything you need to know about what it needs. Learn to listen to its cues. Here are some signals that your body is asking you to work in:

⮑ Your breathing is erratic

⮑ You're mentally unfocused or feel out of control

⮑ You're finding it difficult to maintain a broad perspective

⮑ You're "going through the motions" and not really getting the benefit out of your workouts

⮑ You feel like you've hit a performance plateau

⮑ Your workouts are adding to your everyday stress rather than helping you to manage it

⮑ You find it difficult to wind down even when the opportunity for rest presents itself

⮑ You feel exhausted yet you are having trouble sleeping

When in doubt, don't be afraid to err on the side of rest. Trust yourself to start recognizing these signs as invitations to work in and you will sharpen your intuition and your ability to be more flexible in your approach, which will serve you well in all your pursuits.

We're so busy that we marginalize recovery and keep putting it off, quarantining it to the off-season or rest days rather than prioritizing and normalizing it as a critical daily occurrence. So it shouldn't be a surprise that even when you do have the opportunity to rest, relaxation can feel elusive. If tension lingers long after your workout is over, or if you find yourself lying awake at night with your mind abuzz, you're well aware of this all-too-common scenario. You have to intentionally calm your nervous system in order to shift from effort to ease—from SNS engagement to PNS response. Use your nervous system to full advantage to optimize your recovery. Now more than ever, optimal recovery requires tangible skills, practice, and diligence—it requires you to work in.

When I Do Stop, What Should I Do?

Once you learn to listen to your body, how do you effectively transition from working out to not working out in order to make the best use of downtime and rest days? How do you ensure productive recovery? How do you recover for real? Working in equips you with two key skill sets to accomplish this:

1

MENTAL FOCUS TRAINING

2

PHYSICAL RELAXATION PRACTICE

Recovery is personal. And despite any beliefs you have about its place in your training and life, consider the fact that it doesn't have to be confined to evenings or weekends or vacations. It shouldn't be relegated to downtime or your perceived lack thereof. Waiting until you've crossed everything off your to-do list to relax is like running to stand still. In fact, it probably won't ever happen. Don't wait for injury or burnout to force you into recovery mode. Do it now.

GET REAL

So many factors have a significant impact on the recovery process—nutrition, hydration, sleep, and more. Ultimately, it's up to you to understand what your body needs, listen to its cues, and respond accordingly.

Getting clear about where you're at with your restorative input is a great place to start. Then you can begin to chart a tangible plan to work in, in the context of your unique goals.

How do I value recovery?

Is my resistance to recovery a choice or a habit?

How do I feel when I'm not working out? Why is that?

How will working in help me achieve my goals?

Recover in the time that *is* available to you.

LISTEN TO YOUR BODY

It sounds so obvious, but be honest, when's the last time you let yourself off the hook because you were just too tired to execute your training plan? And then didn't feel bad about it? Or have you ever lowered your expectations for what you hoped to accomplish in a day after waking exhausted from a really poor night's sleep?

This is key for knowing when to slow down and deciding when to stop. Everyone says, "Listen to your body." But do you actually do it? Sometimes you have to push through. But sometimes you have to cut yourself some slack—and, more important, be okay with it! You'll make up for it when you can train more efficiently and effectively because you let your body be the boss.

Don't just talk about "listening to your body." *Do it.*

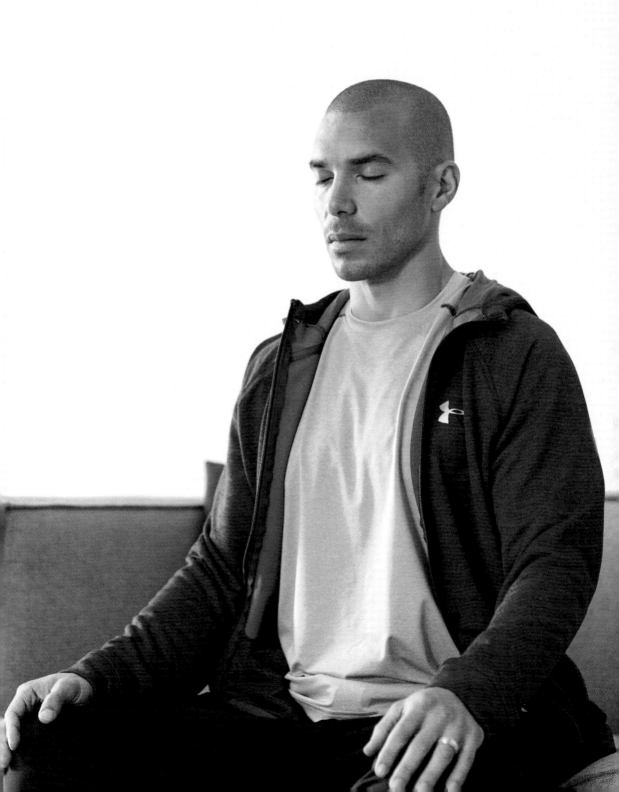

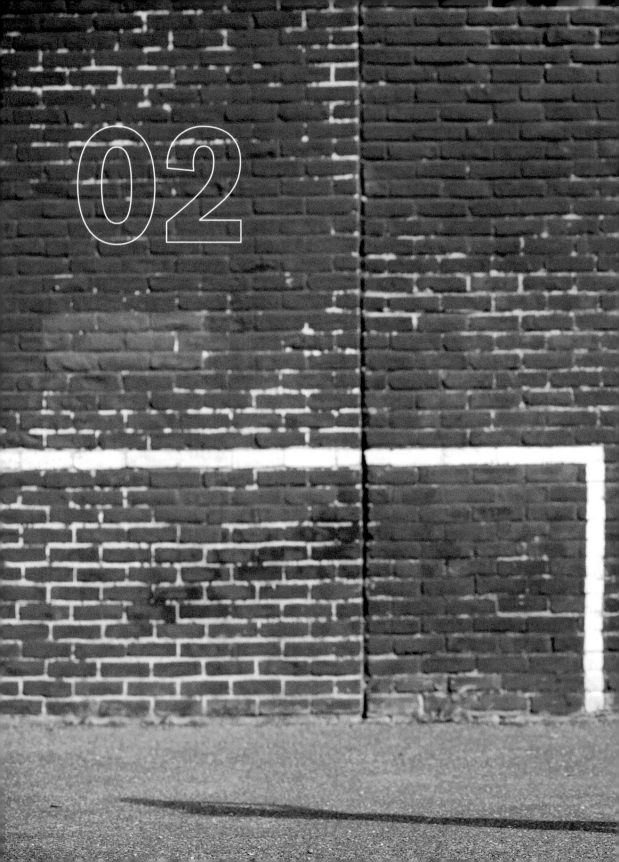

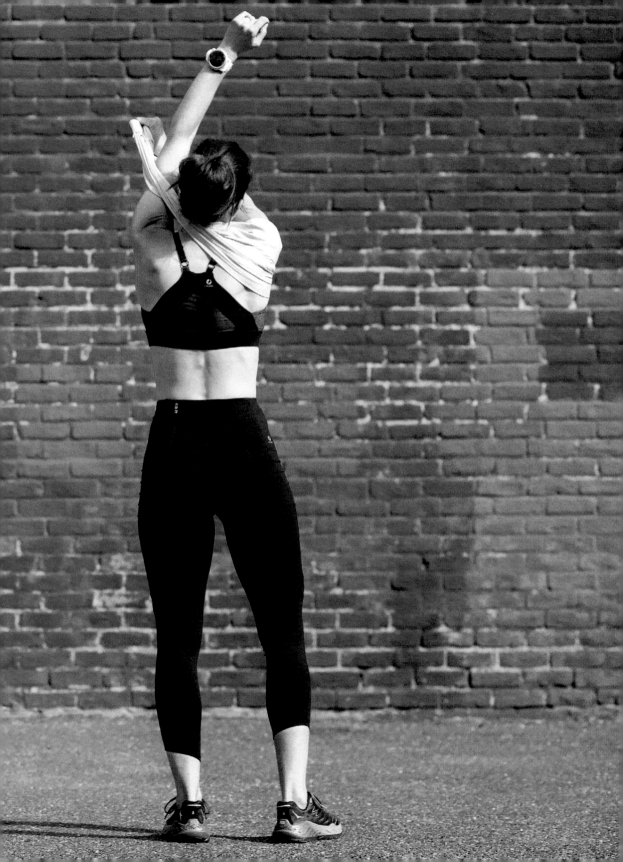

GET YOUR HEAD RIGHT

Meditation is mental focus training that helps us relax and recharge so that we can feel and perform our best in everything we do. It harmonizes our mind and body and gives us more flow—the ability to be fully absorbed in the task at hand—which is as instrumental in resting easy as it is in going hard.

As you go through your workouts and your days, moments of stress accumulate in your mind and body. When left unaddressed, tension builds and makes it more difficult to unwind. It can become pervasive, even normalized, making it more difficult to discern between tension and relaxation—and making real recovery more elusive. That's where meditation comes in.

TENSION = Mental and/or physical strain
that impedes the mind or body

You're probably aware that your mental game is just as important as your physical prowess. Your mind is naturally your most powerful asset, and, like your muscles, it gets stronger when you train hard. But don't miss out on the chance to build mental resilience after your workout is done.

You need mental strength to focus on what's happening and to keep going. It requires clear resolve to let go of your memories, thoughts, and projections, and embrace the moment you are in. Athletes—like most people—are so accustomed to planning and problem-solving that it can be unfamiliar and

Reach as far inward as you do outward.

uncomfortable to slow the constant race of thoughts, let alone quiet it, even if you like the idea of a mental break and believe that you would benefit from it. When your workout gets hard you keep putting out more effort because you're used to it—you practice all the time. You can apply the same determination to recovery and keep putting in more ease even when it feels hard—and maximize results on both ends of the spectrum as a result. But you have to practice.

Why Meditate?

You know your mind is powerful. Since the beginning of time people have sought ways to focus the mind and harness its power. And while historical contexts of mental focus might conjure images of monks chanting on mountainsides, today people are meditating on everything from their worries to their goals in order to gain clarity and get results, and athletes are using meditation to get an edge. Recent research has made the benefits of regular meditation undeniable, and people are bending traditional techniques to fit their modern lifestyles.

MEDITATE = To focus your mind on something

Now focus—meditate—on this: Applying the same mental focus to your recovery that you do to your workouts will not only improve the results of your recovery but also yield better results from your workouts. If you're serious about your goals you should care about meditation because it will help you work in. It's a restorative shifting of your perspective that signals to your internal systems that the props that help you meet and overcome challenges can let go so that you can transition back into a more relaxed state where effort can be fully absorbed. Meditation helps you to deliberately rest after a sweat session, allowing you to make the most of your recovery time.

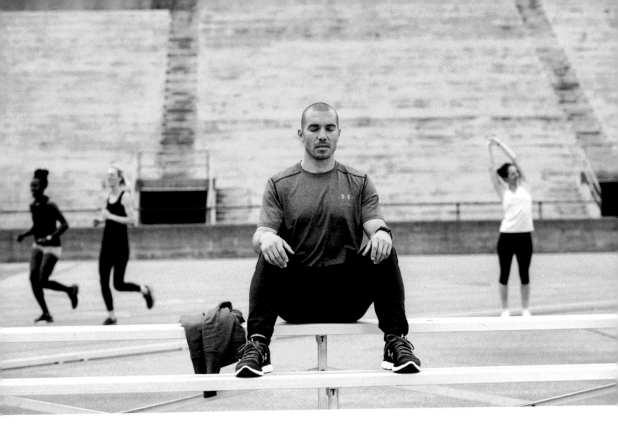

In sport and life, meditation helps you:

FOCUS. Meditation sharpens mental focus and concentration. We spend a lot of time rehashing the past and projecting into the future. When you meditate, you bring your attention into the present moment—which is where optimal experiences exist and where recovery is optimized.

MANAGE PHYSICAL PAIN. Meditation calms your nervous system and eases residual tension, which is incredibly helpful for managing physical pain.

INCREASE EMOTIONAL STABILITY. Meditation's calming effects help manage anxiety and depression. It helps you to stay connected to your goals and to keep perspective even when confronted with life's inevitable challenges and adversity.

TRANSCEND UNPRODUCTIVE HABITS. Everyone has deeply ingrained habits—the behaviors you default to subconsciously that sometimes act as coping mechanisms—

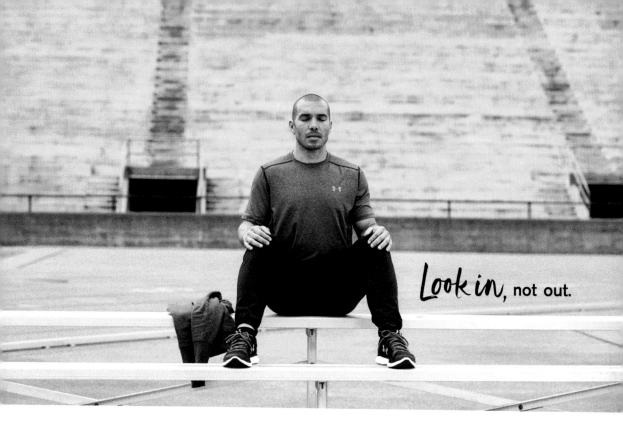

Look in, not out.

based on your usual mode of operation. Meditation helps you become aware of these habits, especially the ones that are not serving you, so you can begin to determine more productive possibilities.

STRENGTHEN YOUR IMMUNE SYSTEM. By calming your nervous system and shifting you into a more relaxed state, meditation gives your immune system a well-deserved break before you get run down.

IMPROVE SLEEP. Meditating is an ideal transition to a restful night's sleep because it creates space between your work and your rest.

There's more. You know those times when you are totally engaged, yet completely relaxed, and even effort seems effortless—people often describe this feeling as "flow." This state, where ability and enjoyment are optimized, doesn't have to be as elusive as it might seem. Meditation gives you the ability to deliberately find more flow any-time, anywhere, rather than waiting for the planets to seemingly align in your favor.

As an athlete, this skill is invaluable when you need to get in the zone at game time. But you also need to seek flow after the clock stops because the ability to intentionally relax optimizes recovery, which in turn supercharges all your output.

FLOW = To be fully absorbed in the task at hand

Or maybe this scenario is familiar: You've done your workout, you're totally wiped out, and you're ready to relax. But your body remains abuzz and your mind continues

---

MEDITATION IS AN INPUT

"But my run is my meditation," you say? Beyond the physical benefits of running, you probably enjoy it because it "fills you up" or fuels you in some way. While a great run might feel meditative or restorative, it doesn't yield the same recovery benefits as a meditation in stillness. Here's why:

→ Many people exercise to relieve stress. Physical activity helps you to get out of your head—it shifts your focus away from perceived stressors—by pulling your attention into your body and the physical task at hand. It literally helps you to shake off stress. While this usually feels refreshing, don't make the mistake of using more and more exercise simply as a break or distraction from stressors, and don't confuse the relief you feel from shifting gears as recovery. Running is by definition an output.

→ You might take pride in your ability to get up and go from 0 to 60, but things don't naturally flow in the opposite direction when you're done training. You can't go from 60 to 0 instantaneously. Your mind and body need space to unwind—a pause between activities—in order to make an effective transition to the task at hand and ease residual stress and tension. Meditation helps to create that space between your work and your rest, no matter how busy you are. Meditation in stillness makes space for input.

to race. You're still amped up. You do a couple of quick stretches. You eat a bar and a banana. You try to take a nap. But you continue to feel a hum, a charge, a sense of energy pulsing through your body. You can't get into a restorative flow so you go through the motions of "recovery" without actually feeling relaxed, and it's frustrating. This isn't real recovery. Rather, it's more doing, as you plow through your post-workout to-do list, which won't help you rejuvenate in a meaningful way.

Flow on Purpose

Try to get your head around this: "How" you are during recovery is the same way you are when you do everything else. Are you easily bored? Or hard on yourself? Do you give up easily? The same could probably be said for how you are when you work out—it's a mirror of your usual way of being. If you tend to react negatively and get down about things not going as planned on your run, like when you don't nail your paces or you get a side stitch, you might discover similar reactions to unexpected happenings during recovery, like when you are struggling to let go of your to-do list or your kid won't stop jumping on you. How resilient are you in the face of real challenges? How calm and unaffected can you be? Observing what comes up for you when you face mental challenges while you meditate gives you insight into how you manage adversity on the track, court, or field as well as in life. Meditation slows you down enough—it literally makes you stop—so that you can be aware of your tendencies and decide whether they're productive. Going forward, you can become more discerning about how you behave or respond to what is happening and hopefully maintain a more broad, positive perspective, especially when things don't go your way. Meditation helps you find your flow regardless of the circumstances.

How you are *here* is how you are *everywhere.*

WHERE'S YOUR PENDULUM?

Meditation helps you to more accurately assess your energy levels. Imagine that your energy is like a pendulum, which should constantly swing between input and output. When you meditate, you become more aware of where that pendulum actually is so that when it swings too far in one direction, or for too long, you can more consciously swing it back in the other direction preemptively—before you get run down, burned out, or worse, injured.

- Visualize a pendulum swinging side-to-side. Output, or effort, swings it to one side and input, or ease, swings it to the other.

- Notice where your energy is right now—how far has the pendulum swung in one direction?

- And now consider at what point it will swing too far (if it hasn't already), and what will prompt you to proactively guide it back in the other direction, knowing that working out and working in are equally important.

Remember, recovery isn't just about stretching or kicking back on the couch. It's about cultivating the ability to flip the switch from effort to ease—on purpose.

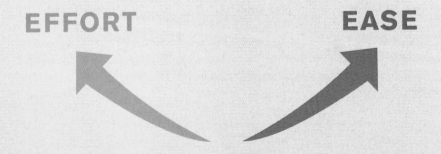

Make the Most of Stress

Stress tends to be generated by our perception of threat to the things we care about, or the sheer volume of things we are trying to manage. When's the last time you felt stressed over something that you're totally indifferent about? Exactly. As athletes, this perception is closely tied to our goals. We are quick to label the surge of chemicals and resulting emotion that accompanies any change related to our goals as stress. While it is likely a reaction to our perception of threat, we hold negative assumptions about it that can trigger a deer-in-the-headlights, "OMG, I'm so stressed," physical tension-inducing downward spiral when things don't go our way or feel beyond our control. Obviously, there are major life events that can be highly stressful and are oftentimes totally out of our control (moving to a new house, losing a job, becoming very ill, etc.), but when daily

WHAT IS CONSCIOUSNESS?

Awareness exists in the present moment, but our typical state of consciousness is oriented around the past or the future. As a result, we blow right past what's happening right here, right now and end up operating unconsciously, or going through the motions of what's happening. For example, if you're tired at the end of a long week but decide to squeeze an extra lifting session in on Friday evening anyway, you might march your body through reps while in your head you're obsessing over the events of the week and organizing your weekend to-do list. Are you getting the full benefit out of your workout? Probably not. How can you if you're merely relying on muscle memory to execute the movements while you're mentally checked out? The sheer volume of life and training today makes it increasingly difficult to train, compete, and live consciously. Luckily, meditation is a tool that can help us to become more self-aware and purposeful in everything that we do—especially recovery. It helps us to do things on purpose rather than defaulting to habit.

CONSCIOUSNESS = Being aware, on purpose

life stress (traffic, commitments, work, etc.)—which is what stress in this context refers to—runs rampant, it steals our energy, productivity, and happiness. And it halts recovery. If you don't address this reality it's likely that you'll be managed by stress rather than it being managed by you. Like a vicious cycle, stress in your life will negatively impact your sports performance, and stress in your sports will negatively impact your life.

Ultimately, it's your outlook or perspective that either keeps you on a positive trajectory or leads you to crash and burn in the presence of challenge or adversity. Stress can feel like a buzzing sensation, or a physical squeeze, or like you are sprinting with no finish line in sight. But in those moments, instead of labeling these observations as negative and allowing yourself to feel overcome, try to acknowledge the reality in front of you and aim to more intentionally relax in order to help shift your perspective and more easefully manage what is actually happening. Doing this will help you harness any chemical surges you are feeling and use them to full advantage. You know what it's like to finish a tough workout and have a heavy workload to dive back into—you might feel stressed before you even untie your running shoes, even though the physical stress of your workout is over. Rather than skimping on working in because you're worried about all there is to do, embrace a pause to calm your mind and body post-workout, knowing that is the top priority regardless of what's next on your agenda.

EASE = Absence of tension

Don't confuse ease and easy—they are not the same thing. While easy is the opposite of hard—implying an absence of difficulty—ease is a relaxed way of being that, marked by an absence of tension, you can apply to any situation, making your desired outcome more likely. The surge of stressful energy you're feeling will still be there after you've had a few moments to relax, but you'll be better able to use it to full advantage to get stuff done, rather than feeling frazzled. Ultimately, ease delivers energy. Meditation will bring you more ease, which will give you more energy. In other words, with practice you might find that meditation is like serving yourself an espresso—without the threat of a caffeine crash. Meditation helps you to sustain the broader perspective needed to cope in a positive, productive manner, no matter what comes at you.

STRESS LESS

Rather than saying "I'm stressed" and allowing yourself to be owned by what is likely a transient reaction to your perception of threat, instead say: "I notice _____ ." Create more space between you and "it" by seeing it rather than being it. See the source of stress as a cloud floating across the sky, trusting that however it is making you feel, it too will pass. This detachment allows you to be more discerning about how to manage what is happening and more easeful in what you do next.

I notice –
see it rather than be it ...
detachment

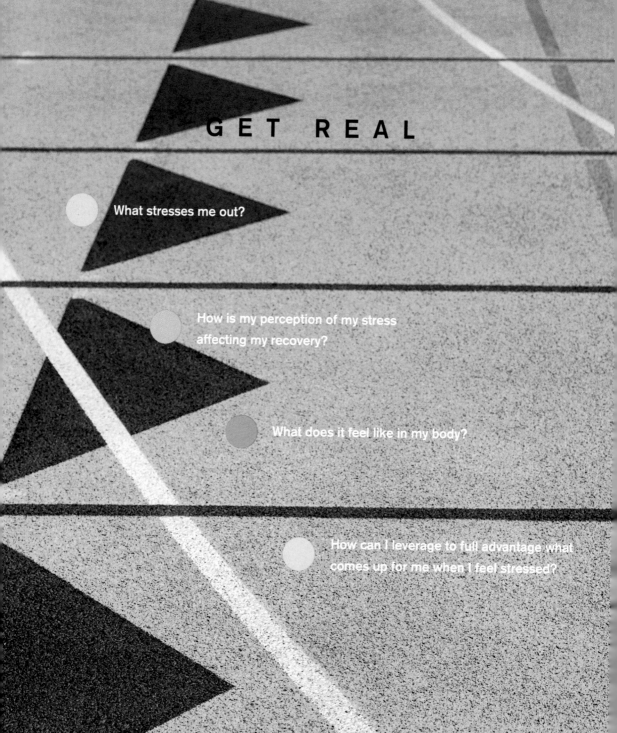

GET REAL

What stresses me out?

How is my perception of my stress affecting my recovery?

What does it feel like in my body?

How can I leverage to full advantage what comes up for me when I feel stressed?

GET REAL

Get real about why you are meditating. Be clear about the purpose of this mental focus training in the context of working in—optimizing your recovery—because that understanding will help to keep you motivated and moving in the right direction.

I meditate because:

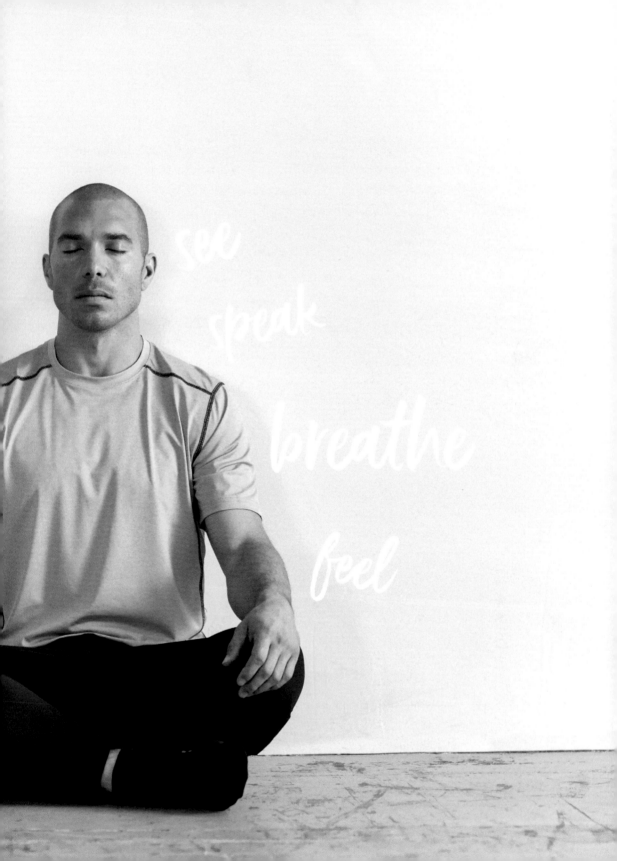

How to Meditate

It's how you meditate that matters. Where most athletes go wrong is failing to prioritize the mental aspects of recovery and approaching meditation as a to-do that they have to fit into their already crammed training and life schedule. When approached in a rigid way, meditation ends up more forced than fluid, and you'll be less likely to make it a consistent part of your routine and more likely to think it doesn't work and so give up.

Instead, aim to clock as little as 2 focused minutes as a real break and buffer between the activities of your day, between your work and your rest. Consider it an oasis during the busiest of days or training cycles, giving you the strength and resilience you need to win at whatever you're doing. Think of it as a chance to recharge and reconnect to your goals and the person who is most instrumental in achieving them: you. Use meditation to literally relax back into yourself. Start by doing it for yourself, and experience the difference it makes. Before long, you'll be doing it for enjoyment because, like anything, when you approach it with enthusiasm it will be more fun. You'll also get more out of it.

The Tools

One of the best things about meditation is that you can do it anytime, anywhere, and you already possess all the tools you need to do it effectively. When you practice, you will probably notice that it's hard to think about nothing. Without a clear focal point, your mind is likely to wander. Luckily, your innate tools give your mind something to wrap itself around, helping to anchor your attention in what's happening right here, right now, which is the key to successful meditation and ultimately real recovery. Use each of these highly portable tools like a GPS during meditation to guide you back into yourself anytime.

BREATHE. Your breath is your most powerful, accessible tool to activate relaxation and kick-start the recovery process. Your mind and breath are directly connected. In any given moment, your breathing is a direct reflection of your interior state—it will tell you exactly what you need to know about what's happening inside. Shallow, erratic breathing can raise blood pressure and increase heart rate, as well as send your mind into overdrive; deep, steady breathing helps you to relax and remain steadfast. Most breathing exercises are effective in just a few breaths.

SPEAK. Mantras are positive affirmations that anchor you in the present and cut through any chaos or negativity in your head. You can make them specific to your circumstances and use them to calm your mind and realign yourself with your unique intentions.

SEE. Visualization increases belief in your abilities and can help you harmonize what you think you want and what you believe is possible. Feeling overwhelmed? See yourself becoming calmer as you resolve to do what you can, when you can, productively completing one task at a time. Have an injury? See it healing as you patiently allow that trouble spot to rest and regain balance with help from your PT exercises. Want to achieve a specific goal? See yourself approaching the finish line as you diligently work out and work in. When you visualize yourself achieving your desired outcome by positively, proactively navigating the terrain between your current reality and end goal, you will likely find any fixations or fears about why you "can't" or "aren't progressing" fade into the background. Visualization broadens your perspective. It shifts you into a more positive, easeful state, which by default makes it more likely that you will grasp whatever it is that you have your heart set on.

FEEL. To recover effectively, you need to relax. Once you feel it, you can be it—you are it. Using your awareness to feel into your physical body and consciously release any lingering tension is one of the best ways to do this. Meditation that is anchored to your felt sense helps you to distinguish between tension and relaxation and get it done.

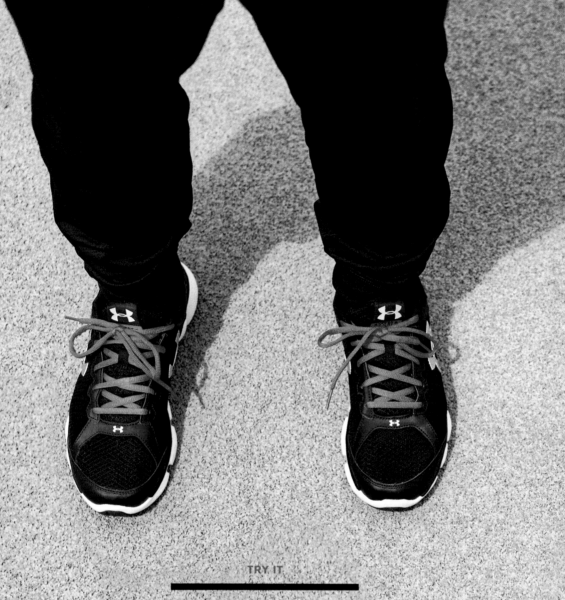

FEEL YOUR FEET

Pause, close your eyes, and feel where your energy is—notice where it is in your body. If you are busy, multitasking, or stressed, it's likely that you feel more sensation, tension, or a buzz in your head, chest, or elsewhere in your upper body. Now focus on your feet and notice how when you deliberately move your focus down your body, it helps you to calm down and feel more grounded.

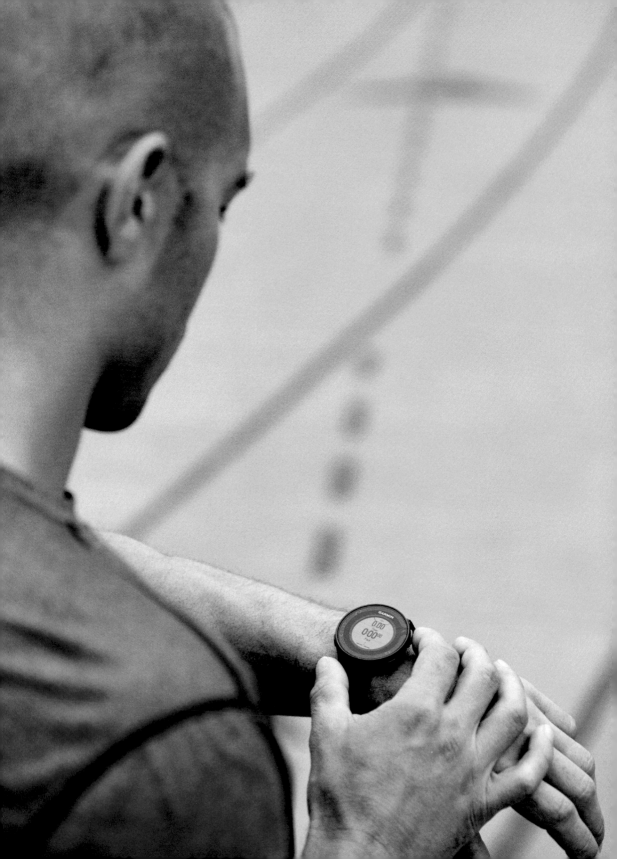

HOW TO GET STARTED

WHEN: Set aside some time to meditate. For recovery purposes, it's ideal to use these practices post-workout or as you wind down your day. That being said, being consistent is key, so practice whenever it best fits into your schedule, which could be different from day to day.

WHAT: Choose a focus for your meditation and select a routine based on how you feel.

DURATION: It doesn't matter whether you have 2 minutes or 20. The key is to make it happen consistently—ideally every day. Longer meditations give you more time to enter a restful state and settle in, so aim to spend as long as possible. But don't skip it altogether if you're short on time. In those instances, embrace whatever time is available as an impactful, restorative pause.

WHERE: Aim for a quiet spot where you can sit comfortably. On the floor next to your bed, sitting tall on your couch, or on a pillow on your living room floor are all good options. If there are distractions around, approach them as an added challenge that will further sharpen your focus and make your practice more real.

BREATHE: Inhale and exhale through your nose, unless otherwise instructed or if you are congested, in which case breathe through your mouth.

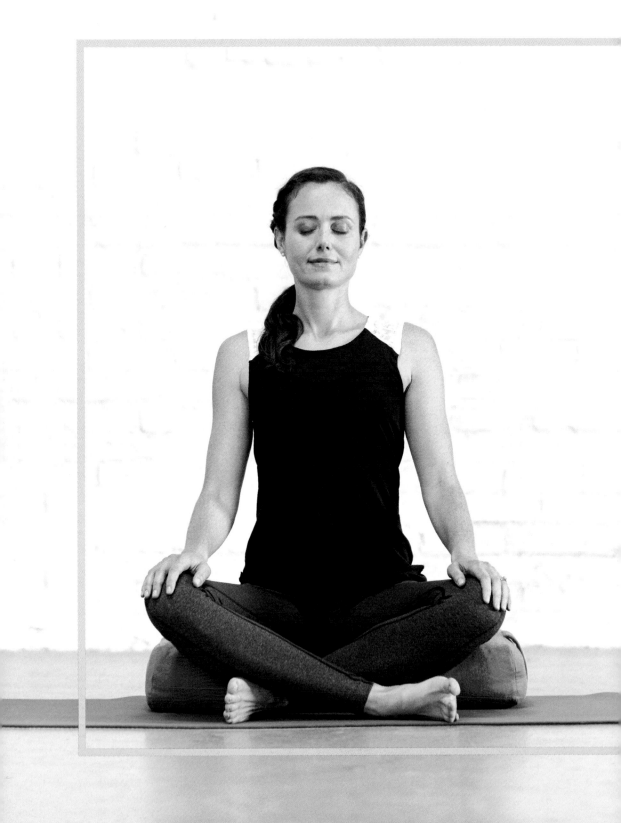

HOW TO SIT

Sitting tall helps to neutralize your spine, which optimizes your posture and breathing. Your body supports your breath and your breath supports your body. But it shouldn't be rigid. Comfort is equally important so that you can more readily focus and lean into relaxation, rather than dying for it to be over. Try these options to find your most comfortable seat, and remember that the more you do it, the more comfortable it will become, the more natural it will feel, and the more readily you will be able to hold yourself in a balanced way, even as you rest:

ON A PROP. Sit on a bolster, pillow, or folded blanket so that your hip flexors relax and you can sit tall. Loosely cross your legs or extend them out in front of you if needed for knee comfort. Rest your hands palms down on your knees or thighs and drop your shoulders down and back.

AT THE WALL. If it feels hard to lengthen your spine tall toward neutral, take your prop (bolster/pillow/blanket) to the wall so you have support to lean into.

IN A CHAIR. If hip or low back discomfort makes sitting on the floor feel like agony, sit tall on the edge of a chair.

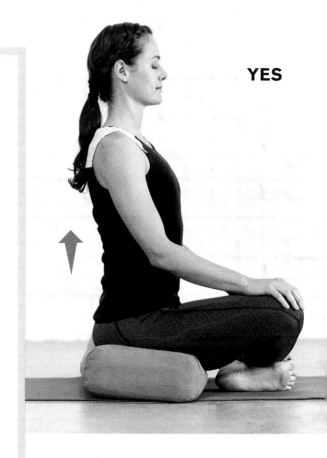

YES

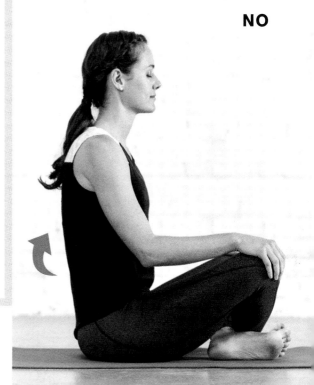

NO

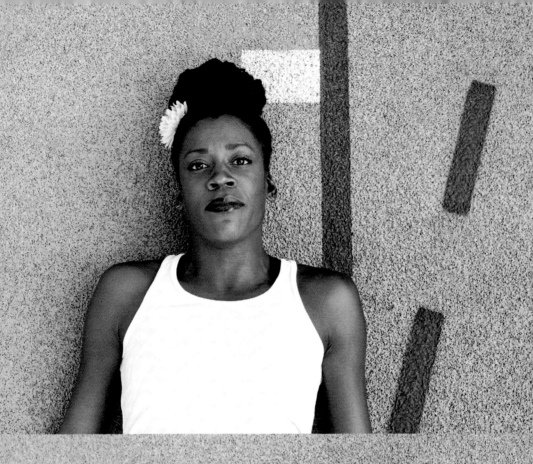

TRY IT

CLOSE YOUR EYES

Slowly close your eyes to create a distinct shift from out to in, from external stimulation to internal experience—which is where real recovery happens.

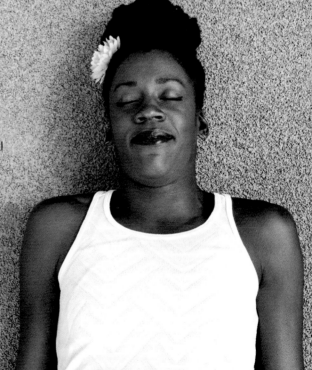

Hurdle the Barriers

Let's be real: It's hard to stop and think about nothing. Rest assured that if you don't feel complete bliss after your first 5 minutes of meditating, it's not because you're not doing it right.

You can't force yourself to relax. Similarly, you can't force meditation. That being said, for meditation to work and make an impact, you can't approach it passively. It's not some flaky thing you can stumble into spontaneously whenever it happens to be convenient.

Meditation isn't easy. But it doesn't have to be so hard.

To harness meditation's restorative superpowers takes commitment. Successful meditation requires the same effort and vigor that you bring to your other training. Just as you push through mental roadblocks when you work out, you'll need to overcome mental barriers when you work in. While you can't muscle your way through working in, you've got to stay with it.

Here are some common meditation challenges and strategies to cope with them:

PHYSICAL DISCOMFORT. Sitting can be uncomfortable. Don't let an achy back or stiff hips put a damper on your meditation mojo. Meditating in a restorative yoga posture can be a good alternative to sitting. And if you need to lie down it's okay! Make sure you're comfortable before you begin so that you can relax into your mental focus training rather than dying for it to be over. Do what you have to do.

LABELING. There's no such thing as "good" or "bad" meditation. There's only you shifting your focus inward and reconnecting to yourself. So scratch "I'm not good at it" off your list of worries and excuses.

PLANNING. What's for dinner? What workouts will I do this weekend? If you're forecasting the future, remind yourself that what is most important in this moment is this meditation, this time you're taking to clear your mind—that is what is going to help you best manage whatever comes next.

DAYDREAMING. Your mind will wander like a dog off its leash. Daydreaming isn't meditating. Notice when your attention has drifted and gently guide it back to what's happening right now.

CLOCK WATCHING. Set a timer before you begin based on how much time you have to meditate. Then detach from duration. Don't wonder "how much longer." You selected a specific duration because that time is available—use it.

DISTRACTIONS. If closing your eyes seems to cue the leaf blowers or your kid is going nuts in the next room, see if you can embrace the noise as "meditation for real" rather than allowing it to wind you up. Face it, there will always be distractions. What matters is how you manage them.

EMOTIONAL DISCOMFORT. When you're still and let go of busyness, sometimes unexpected emotions rise to the surface—feelings that you might perceive as negative in some way. Bravely observe and sit with whatever comes up rather than trying to suppress it; pent-up emotions can be a significant energy drain and deter real recovery.

PROCRASTINATION. When you have free time, you might feel like you need to use it to "get stuff done." You might find yourself saying, "I'll meditate after I do XYZ. . . ." But there will always be stuff to get done. Don't miss out on your opportunity to generate the energy needed to handle whatever tasks feel so important.

LACK OF MOTIVATION. Don't feel bad or give up if you don't feel like meditating. Trust that over time your diligence will generate strong motivation.

DIFFICULTY REMEMBERING ROUTINES. You'll likely find certain approaches or routines more helpful than others. If you struggle to remember how to execute them or simply prefer being guided, try putting on headphones and using a guided meditation—there's a library of options for this at video.jasyoga.com.

Practice!

GET REAL

Don't be discouraged, or feel like you're not doing it right, or that it's a waste of time if you experience hurdles in your meditation practice. Instead realize they are part of the process of building the mental resilience required for real recovery. And, like most things in life, what matters is how you manage challenges productively to get results. If you wait for the perfect time to meditate, it probably won't happen.

The challenges I perceive about meditation are:

When I encounter these scenarios, I feel:

This is how I will overcome them:

When I stay with it, post-meditation feels like:

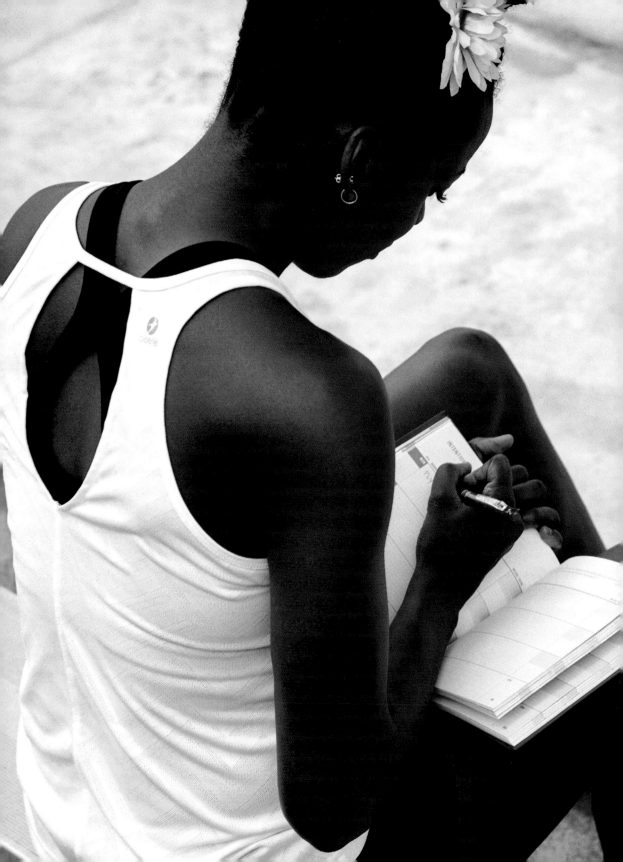

CREATE MORE SPACE FOR RECOVERY

How does rushing around to manage an overbooked schedule feel to you? How does your head feel? And what does busyness feel like in your body? In these times, recovery is usually the first thing to go. But it doesn't have to.

Consider making a more spacious schedule, which is more conducive to consistent, effective recovery. If this feels impossible, that's a good sign you'll benefit immensely from making it a priority to create more space.

If we don't allow for that sense of spaciousness and model that for our teammates, colleagues, and families, no one will.

WORK IN

FOR MENTAL FOCUS

Use these simple routines to help you start meditating, explore different techniques, and ultimately make meditation an integrated daily activity to optimize your recovery. As your familiarity and understanding of these techniques grow, your ability to evolve the practices to suit your specific needs will, too.

GAME PLAN

⇒ Choose a routine and get comfortable.

⇒ Set a timer for however long you want to practice—aim for at least 5 to 10 minutes.

⇒ Pause and notice how you feel; use the pre-/post-game (p. 46).

⇒ Do a routine.

⇒ When the timer ends, pause and feel the difference; use the pre-/post-game again.

⇒ Onward!

Use **THE PLAN: RECOVER FOR REAL** (p. 162), a month-long plan for more inspiration on how to get started.

Don't wait for recovery.

It shouldn't be a spontaneous, accidental occurrence.

WHERE'S YOUR HEAD?

BEFORE YOU PRACTICE: Pause and notice how you feel. These observations give you a baseline for comparison when you're finished, and help you feel the difference.

⇒ What's your breath like? Is it erratic or steady? Shallow or deep?

⇒ What's on your mind? What are you thinking about?

⇒ What do your thoughts, stress, or whatever you might be trying to manage today feel like in your body?

AFTER YOU PRACTICE: Pause and feel the difference. Use the same questions to check in post-meditation. Taking this extra moment is critical because it helps you become more aware of the effects of your practice, absorb the benefits, and feel motivated to continue.

If you don't notice much difference, don't assume you haven't done it right or that it was a waste of time. As you gain experience, the benefits will become more readily accessible.

Trust the process.

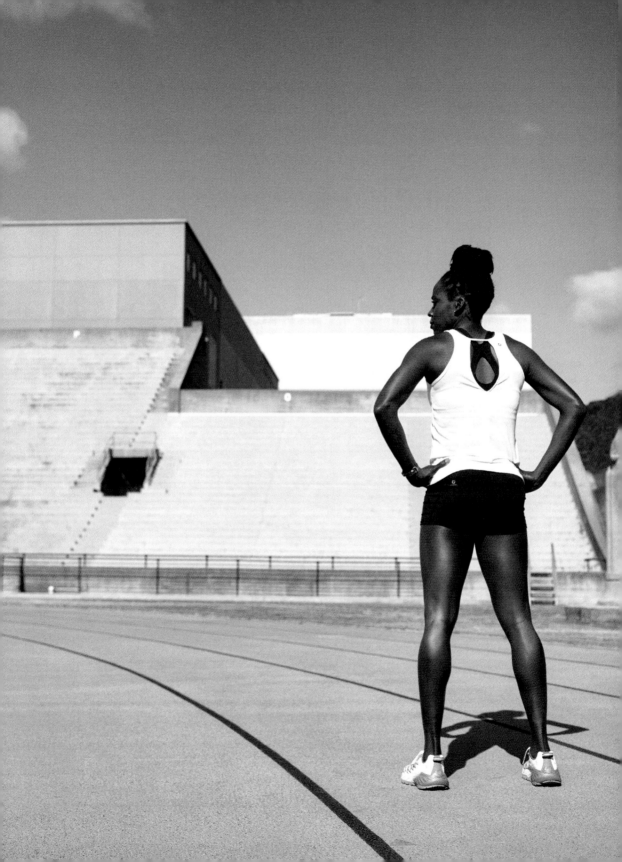

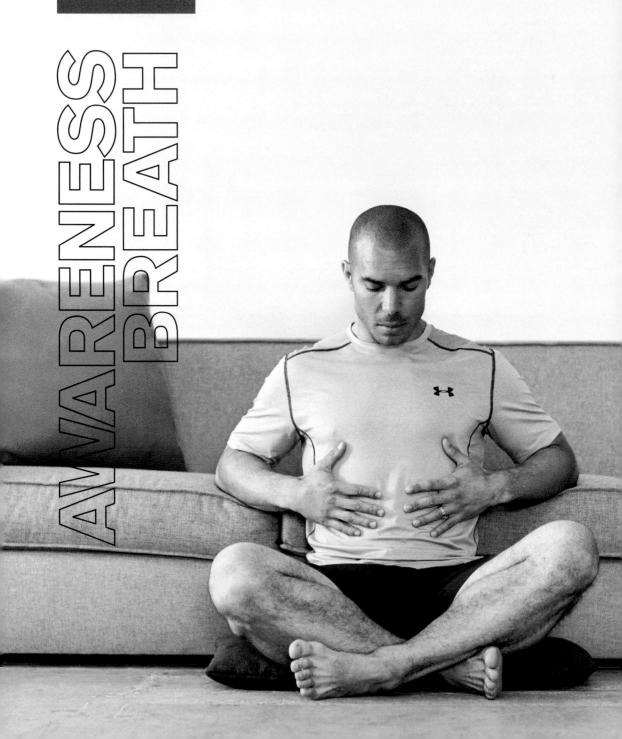

AWARENESS BREATH

WHY

Anchoring your mind to your innate, constant action of breathing is a great way to increase and maintain awareness of your breath so that you can use it to full advantage and sharpen your present moment focus.

HOW

Sit comfortably.

Take a deep breath in . . . a slow breath out.

Continue to deepen your breathing.

Inhaling, say in your head, "I am inhaling . . . "

Exhaling, say, "I am exhaling."

Inhale: "I am inhaling . . . "

Exhale: "I am exhaling."

Continue for several rounds before letting go of the words.

Continue to breathe deeply.

TRY IT

FEEL YOUR BREATH

If feeling your breath from the inside out is elusive, try working from the outside in. Place your hands on your torso and feel your breath lifting and lowering your hands. Move your hands around—to your chest, the sides of your rib cage, your lower abdomen—and keep feeling your breath beneath your hands, which will give you more feedback.

WHY

Lengthening your exhale has a profound calming effect on your nervous system, helping you to slow your heart rate and relax.

HOW

Sit comfortably.

Take a deep breath in . . . a slow breath out.

Continue to deepen your breathing.

Inhale as you count 1–2–3–4.

Exhale as you count 1–2–3–4–5–6.

Breathe in for 4 . . .

And out for 6.

Keep slowing it down, and see if you can lengthen your exhale to 8 or more.

Kick-start recovery with your *breath.*

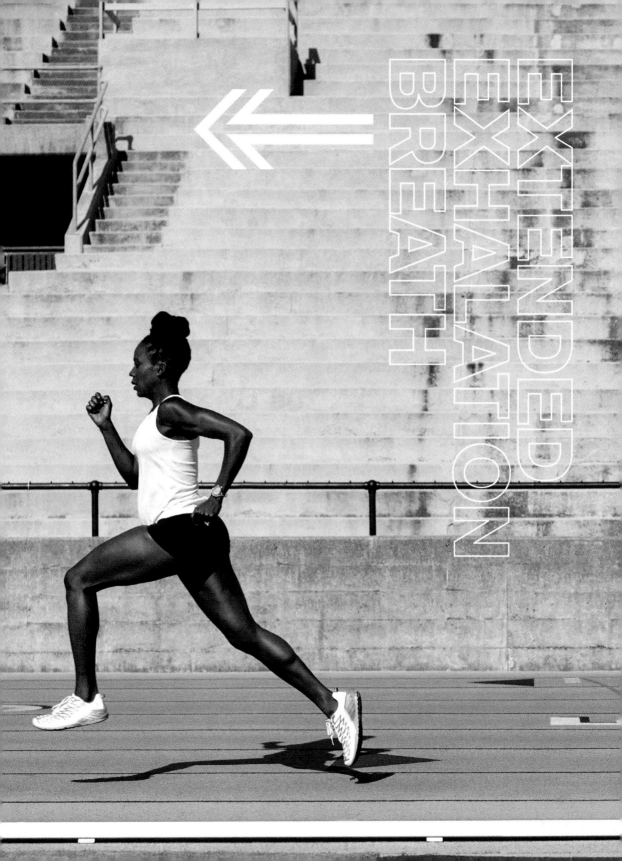

EXTENDED
EXHALATION
BREATH

BELLY BREATH

WHY

When you are tired or stressed, your breath becomes more shallow, making it more difficult to relax. Breathing into your lower abdomen helps to deepen your breath and move your attention downward, which is calming and grounding.

HOW

Sit comfortably.

Take a deep breath in . . . a slow breath out.

Continue to deepen your breathing.

Inhale, inflating your belly as you focus on your lower abdomen, before allowing the breath to fill your chest.

Exhale, relaxing your belly completely.

Continue.

MEDITATION
+YOGA

Couple your meditation with a restorative yoga posture, or do it to begin or end your restorative yoga routine.

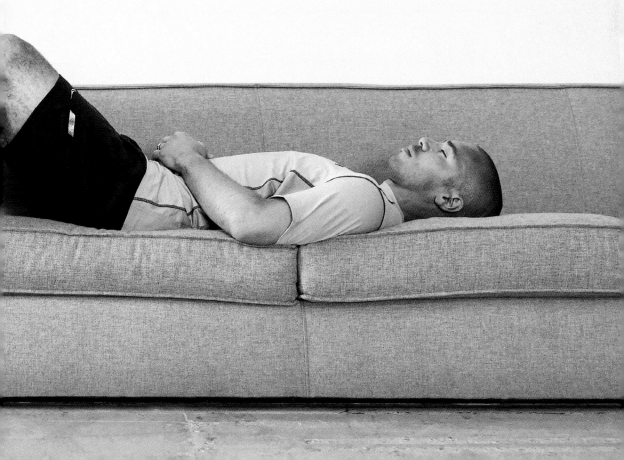

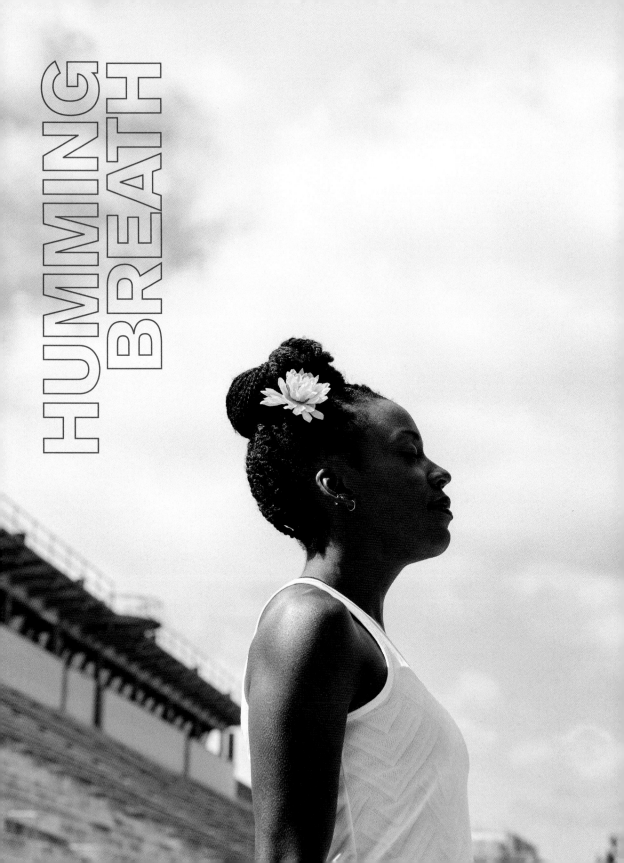

HUMMING BREATH

WHY

Humming creates a vibration in your body that is meditative and calming.

HOW

Sit comfortably.

Take a deep breath in . . . a slow breath out.

Continue to deepen your breathing.

Inhale through your nose.

Exhale through your nose and make a bee-like hum, prolonging your exhale as long as you comfortably can (you shouldn't be left gasping for air).

Again, inhale smoothly . . .

Exhale, hum.

Continue, keeping the volume gentle.

TRY IT

LAY DOWN YOUR TO-DO LIST

Before you meditate, take a moment to acknowledge that you will remember what you need to know or do, and trust that you'll be able to attend to it more effectively when your meditation is done.

MANTRA MEDITATION

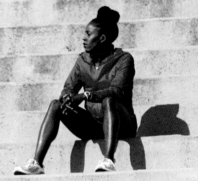

I can rest. I am calm.

WHY

Your favorite mantra or positive affirmation provides a great focal point for meditation, helping to anchor you in the present and bridge the gap between how you feel right now and how you want to feel. Default to a restorative mantra to help you wind down and relax any time.

HOW

Select your mantra, ideally one that is relevant for recovery. For example, "I can rest. I am calm."

Sit comfortably.

Take a deep breath in . . . . a slow breath out.

Continue to deepen your breathing.

Inhaling, say in your head, "I can rest."

Exhaling, say, "I am calm."

Inhale: "I can rest."

Exhale: "I am calm."

Continue.

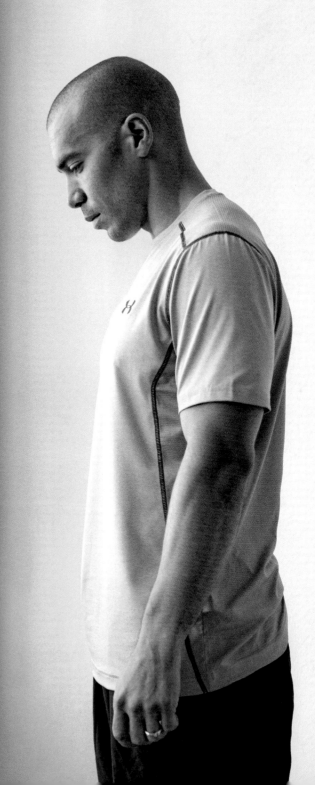

MANTRA
COUNTING

WHY

This technique balances your breathing to calm your nervous system, and your accompanying counting creates a mantra-like meditative quality.

HOW

Sit comfortably.

Take a deep breath in . . . a slow breath out.

Continue to deepen your breathing.

Inhale as you count 1–2–3–4.

Hold as you count 1–2–3–4.

Exhale as you count 1–2–3–4.

Breathe in for 4.

Hold for 4.

Breathe out for 4.

Keep slowing it down, and see if you can lengthen your count to 5 or 6, or more.

WHY

Repeating your mantra to the rhythm of your pulse helps connect your mind and body as you enter a meditative state.

HOW

Sit comfortably and hold your right wrist in your left hand, placing your left thumb on your inner right wrist so that you can feel your pulse.

Take a deep breath in . . . a slow breath out.

Continue to deepen your breathing and feel your pulse beneath your thumb.

Say in your head "I" on one pulse beat . . .

And "am" on the next pulse beat.

Continue to repeat "I am" to the rhythm of your pulse.

Don't force any particular breath pattern or pace—just breathe deeply.

Continue with this mantra, or insert your own—ideally one that is relevant for recovery.

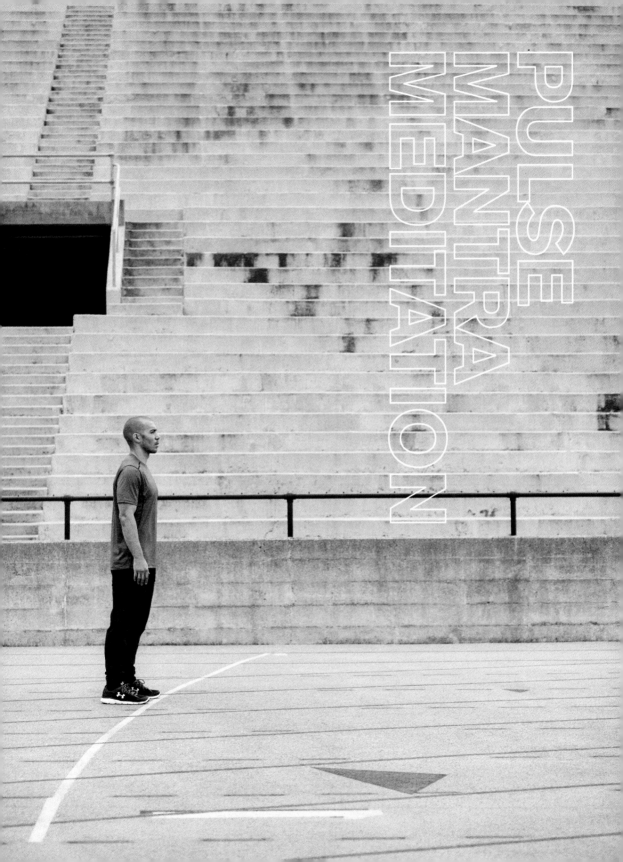

PULSE MANTRA MEDITATION

LET GO

VISUALIZATION

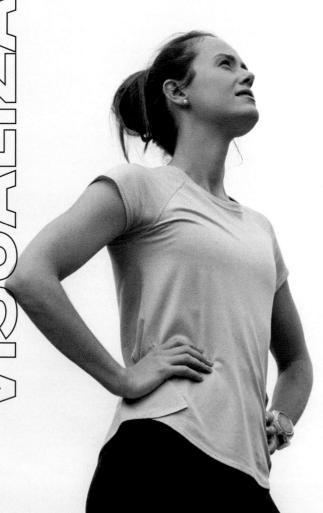

WHY

It's easy to focus on what didn't go right and to beat yourself up about it, which perpetuates habitual tension holding and impedes the recovery process. Instead, acknowledging what has happened and seeing yourself learning from it helps you to let it go and relax, and to recover and grow.

HOW

Sit comfortably.

Take a deep breath in . . . a slow breath out.

Continue to deepen your breathing.

Recall a task or interaction today where you feel you might have fallen short. Be specific about what happened and the feeling it left you with.

Rather than being hard on yourself about it, relax and see the situation as a lesson learned about how you want to handle things next time—visualize yourself behaving in the manner you are most proud of.

Notice how the way you feel about that situation softens, and your body follows.

Now, let go. See yourself as you are right now, stronger for what has happened so that you can be content and relax in this moment in preparation for whatever comes at you next.

Set your sight on how you want to be.

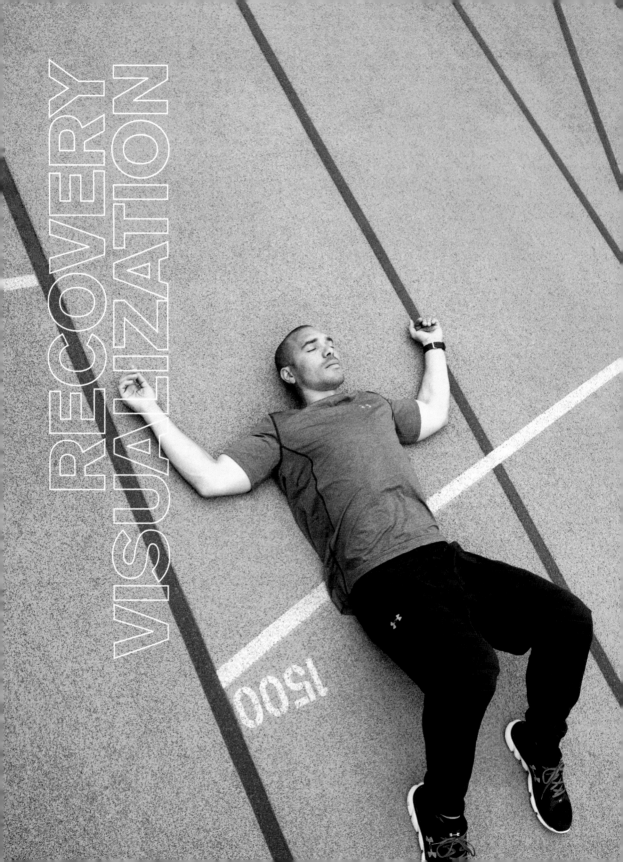

WHY

If you are feeling resistance to giving recovery your full focus, remember that this is likely an unconscious habit rather than a choice. Especially in the times when you are struggling to transition from effort to ease, stop "trying" so hard to relax and use visualization to help you get to the root of the resistance and dissolve it.

HOW

Sit comfortably.

Take a deep breath in . . . a slow breath out.

Continue to deepen your breathing.

Scan your body and notice where any physical resistance to relaxation is happening.

Visualize those specific spots in whatever way they feel—like a tight fist or a diver paralyzed in fear, unable to leap off the diving board; conjure up a specific visual that illustrates that particular tension.

Now take that visual in the opposite direction. See the softening—see the palm opening, see yourself diving into your recovery, by choice, free from anything holding you back.

Continue to identify any lingering resistance, being as specific as possible.

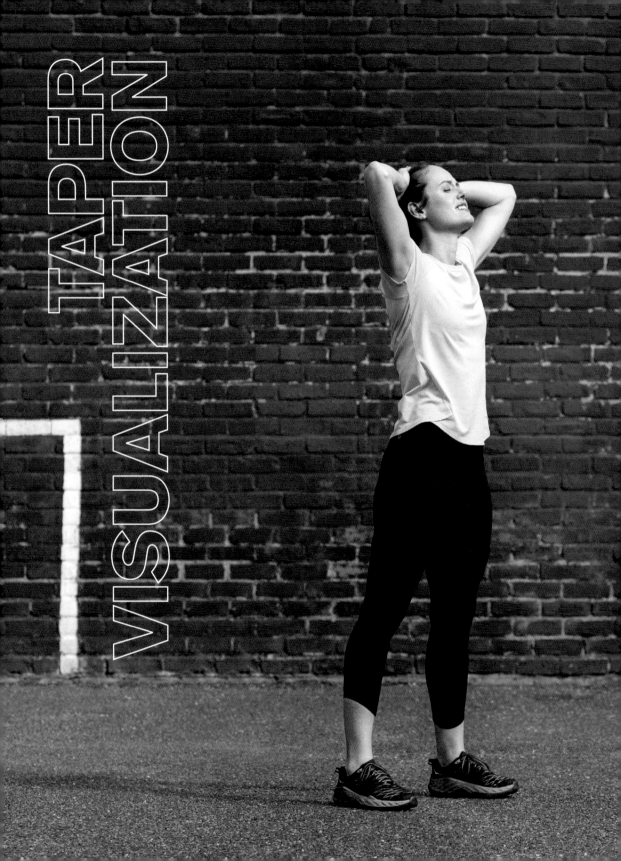

TAPER
VISUALIZATION

WHY

Taper time—when you wind down your workouts to gather your energy and strength for competition—can be a confusing space to navigate. That's why "taper tantrums" are common and pose a very real challenge for many athletes. Visualization can help you embrace and smooth this important transition as you prepare to toe the line.

HOW

Sit comfortably.

Take a deep breath in . . . a slow breath out.

Continue to deepen your breathing.

As you settle in, do a little scan through your training. Be specific as you recap. Notice the moments that stand out—your effort, grit, and perseverance. See them in your mind's eye.

Now, bravely endeavor in the opposite direction.

Trust your hard work and see it settling more deeply into your body as you relax so that it can be optimized.

Now briefly scan your physical body—become aware of any lingering tension and consciously release it.

Continue to trust your training and embrace the taper process.

FEELING MEDITATION

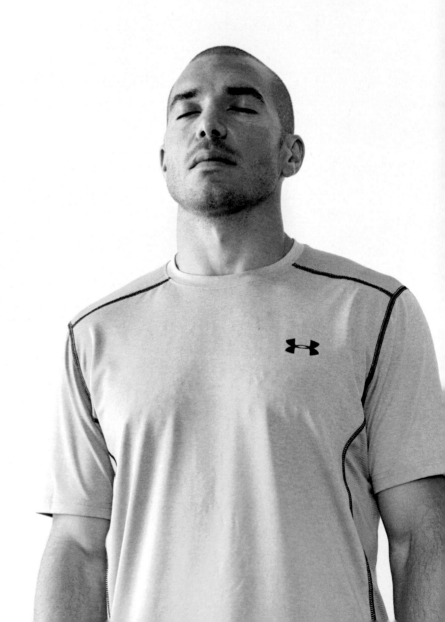

WHY

Bringing your focus to the distinct sensations of your breath entering and exiting your nose helps to add a more tangible, tactile quality to your breathing and ultimately to your meditation.

HOW

Sit comfortably.

Take a deep breath in . . . a slow breath out.

Without trying to force any particular pattern, pace, or depth, become more aware of your breathing. Just breathe.

With your mouth gently closed, focus on your nostrils and notice the sensations of your breath entering and leaving your nose.

Without trying to change anything, continue to feel your breath as you inhale and exhale.

If you become distracted, bring your attention back to the tactile sensations of your breath moving through your nostrils.

Continue.

DISSOLVE TENSION MEDITATION

WHY

"Feeling" your body from the inside out helps you become aware of lingering tension so that you can intentionally release it.

HOW

Sit comfortably.

Take a deep breath in . . . a slow breath out.

Continue to deepen your breathing.

Slowly scan your body, starting with your toes and moving all the way to your head, noticing any lingering tension or stiffness or stress (or whatever word best describes the sensations you feel), and intentionally relax those spots as you go.

Repeat three times, relaxing more and more each time.

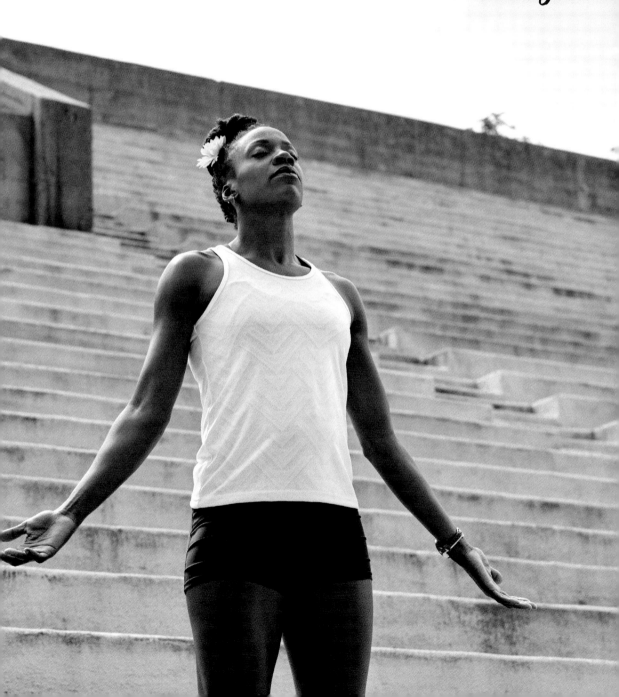

Get out of your *thinking mind* and into your *feeling body*.

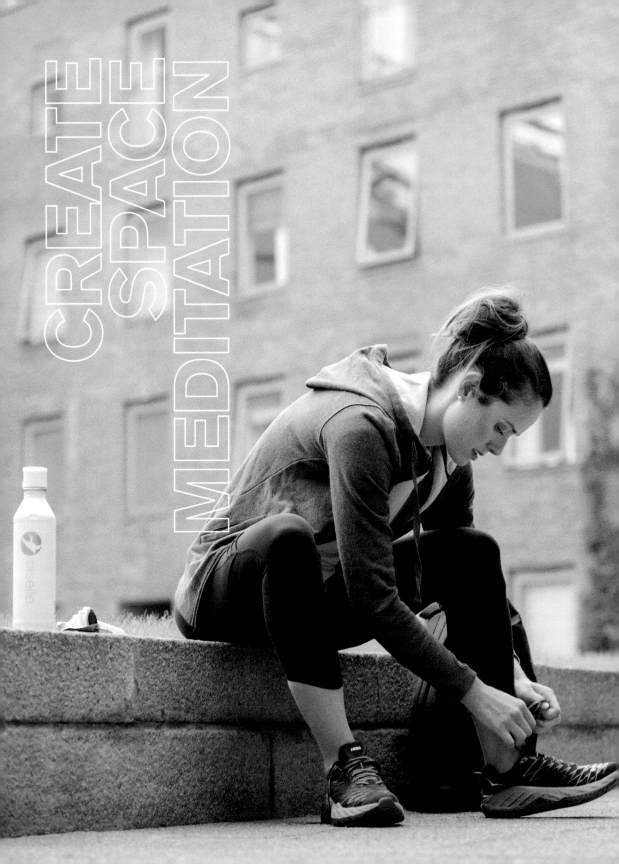

WHY

At the end of the day, and even between activities, it's important to create some space between your work and your rest. When the work or workout is done, don't rush to the next thing. Instead, slow down significantly. Put more space between each one of your thoughts to slow things in your head and more easefully transition through the events of your day. A brief pause will help to ease any lingering tension so that you can be more present for what's up next and, more important, improve the quality of your rest and recovery.

HOW

Sit comfortably.

Take a deep breath in . . . a slow breath out.

Continue to deepen your breathing.

Once your breath feels steady, inhale deeply and hold your breath for a moment, holding only one thought with that breath.

Exhale slowly, letting that thought go.

Again, inhale deeply, perhaps with a different thought . . . hold, then exhale, letting it go and moving on to the next.

Continue, with just one thought per breath, creating and feeling more space as you breathe.

WHY

For those times when you feel overheated mentally and physically, this tactile, meditative breathing technique literally creates a cooling sensation in the body, which helps elicit your relaxation response.

HOW

Take a deep breath in . . . a slow breath out.

Continue to deepen your breathing.

Breathe in through a rolled tongue or through slightly parted lips as if you were drinking from a straw.

Breathe out through your nose.

Continue, feeling the cooling sensation of your breath entering through your mouth, and warm air exiting through your nose.

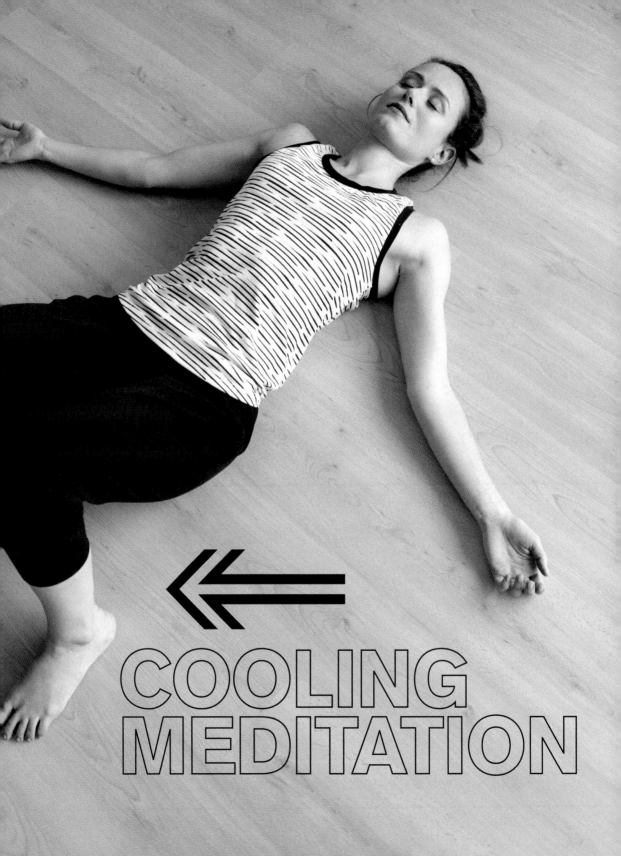

COOLING MEDITATION

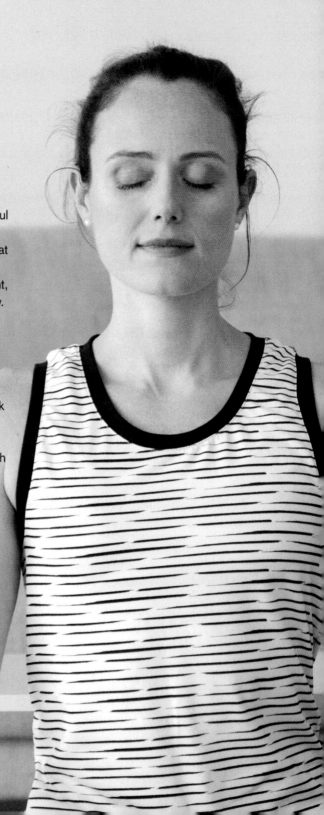

THE 2-MINUTE RESET

When it comes to recovery, anything is better than nothing when you are purposeful in your approach. And luckily, you can meditate anytime, anywhere. While it's great if you have a set daily routine that includes ample time in a distraction-free environment, that's not always possible—and that's okay.

Put it into practice with a 2-minute reset. For example, mornings can be hectic, but you can still use meditation in a meaningful way and set yourself up for a more successful day. While you're waiting for your coffee to brew or your oats to cook in the microwave, stop, sit, and breathe deeply for 2 minutes.

You might find yourself thinking through your to-do list for the day—or notice that the time goes so quickly you wonder if it makes a difference. The more consistently you sit for those 2 minutes, the more efficient you'll become at relaxing and recharging, whether at the start or end of your day.

Anything is better
than nothing.

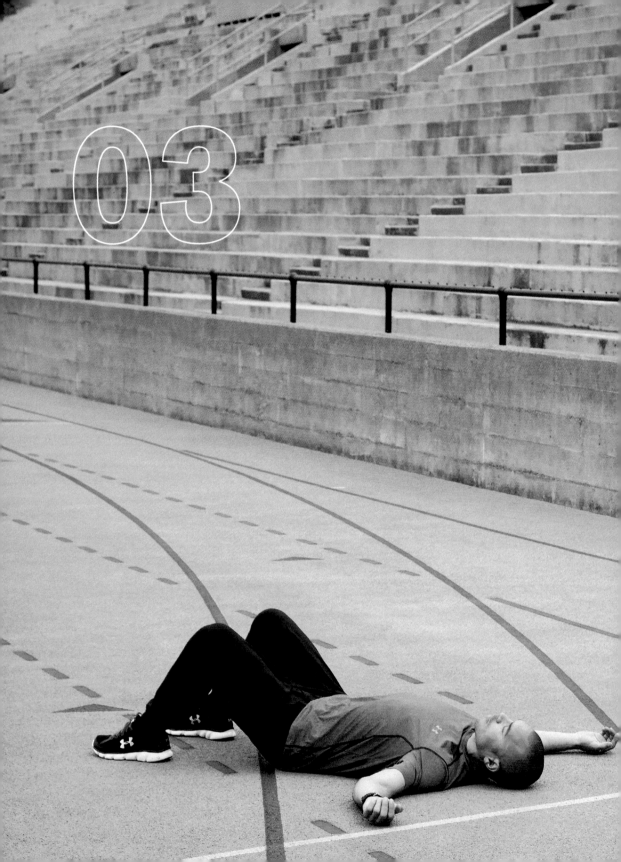

RECHARGE YOUR BODY

Restorative yoga is a physical relaxation practice that calms your body and mind. It's a restful approach to yoga that encourages deep relaxation and promotes physical and mental recovery.

Bear in mind that when it comes to using yoga to achieve your athletic goals, not all yoga is created equal. You work out plenty. The last thing you need is for yoga to be just another workout. But it's not surprising that athletes tend to approach yoga practice as an exploration of their physical limits, which they equate with their capacity to push themselves. When you bring this mind-set to your yoga mat you risk doing more harm than good—because taxing an already exhausted body is likely to work against your training and increase your risk of injury and burnout. Instead, yoga should be used as a tool to retreat from athletic training in order to effectively recharge. When approached in this way it serves as preventative medicine.

Why Do Restorative Yoga?

Restorative yoga aids recovery—it's a legit way to work in—and as a result optimizes athletic potential and performance. Not all yoga has to be restorative to move you toward your goals, but to work in, it does. Restorative yoga is not like other kinds of yoga—it is by definition restful. So if you find yourself doing traditional sun salutations or other dynamic movements in a "restorative" session, know that you are in the wrong place.

When you work out, your body contracts. Muscle fibers shorten as they power your movement. While dynamic stretching is helpful for maintaining flexibility and range of motion, applying force—too much, too hard, too fast—can overwhelm tired muscles, and they will fight you back.

Restorative yoga is a path of less resistance. It helps you open your body with simple postures, often supported by props, that are held longer than in typical yoga classes. Props do the work of supporting your body so that your aching muscles don't have to. And long holds give your body ample time to endeavor in the opposite direction of the status quo. This practice also uses gentle movements to help restore fluidity to muscles, tissues, and joints. The combination of stillness and movement helps your body transition from working to resting, from contraction to expansion.

OPEN = Create space

Don't feel for a big "stretch" like the sensation you might be accustomed to when you reach to touch your toes; you probably won't find it in restorative yoga, and that's okay. Unlike many styles of yoga, the goal of restorative yoga isn't to stretch or strengthen. While some of the poses do indeed stretch your muscles, it's more likely that your connective tissue is being stretched. Imagine you have an internal wetsuit on that surrounds all your muscles and other tissues. Stretching it increases circulation and opens the body in a way that is conducive to deep relaxation and real recovery.

CONNECTIVE TISSUE = Tissue that connects
everything beneath your skin

Restorative yoga optimizes recovery by:
⇒ Decreasing tension
⇒ Increasing breath capacity
⇒ Increasing circulation
⇒ Increasing blood flow to internal organs
⇒ Improving immune system functioning

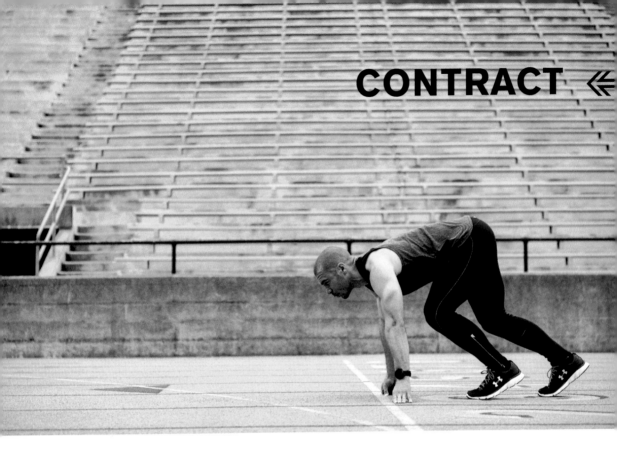

CONTRACT ⇐⇐

It might look easy to lie down on some pillows for 5 minutes, but don't be fooled by the lack of action. You may not be moving, but that doesn't mean nothing is happening or it's an unproductive waste of time. You don't have to physically exert yourself to open your body in restorative yoga because the prop-supported postures do that for you. Think of it as enabling ease.

While you can't force yourself to relax, mindlessly — unconsciously — approaching recovery is unproductive. The effort of restorative yoga is more mental than physical, which in many ways makes it more akin to meditation. For many athletes, there's nothing more difficult than being still. It can be disorienting and agitating to deviate from your usual pace even when you've slowed down on purpose. So you might default to distraction. But if you don't give physical restorative activities your full attention when you're doing them, you won't get the most out of them.

It's difficult to fully address the common lingering tension that impedes the recovery process if you're not even fully aware it's there because you're having a conversation while you're foam rolling or because you skip post-workout stretching in favor of lying

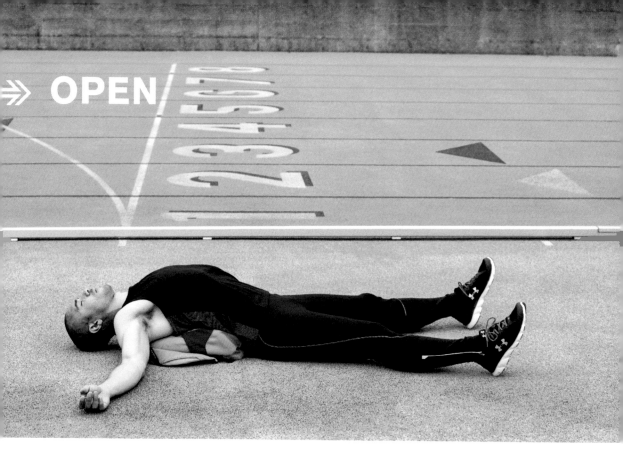

OPEN

on the couch and watching TV. Getting distracted by external stimuli dampens your awareness of your body, impeding your ability to activate recovery in a meaningful way. You might already be aware of this reality and yet still find it difficult to commit to attending to your body's post-workout needs. That's probably because your habit is to do the opposite. And it's not easy.

Restorative yoga can pose some unexpected challenges:
⇒ Boredom
⇒ Frustration
⇒ Unfamiliar and/or uncomfortable physical sensations
⇒ Unexpected emotions

When you are still and paying attention to how your body feels, you might notice that you are a lot more tired or tense or sore (or whatever word best describes it for you) than you realized. This information can be alarming, and you may not know what do with it.

While these challenges aren't that different from what you'll likely encounter when you meditate, you might find that the temptation to multitask is stronger when you are doing physical practices instead of mental ones. For example, you might feel bored in a yoga posture and decide to scroll social media while you rest, whereas you probably wouldn't consider multitasking with devices while you've set a timer for a short meditation, even if your mind starts to wander.

The best way to manage these challenges is to become aware of what comes up for you in these moments of stillness, and to stay with it. Don't back down. Workouts are all about persisting even when you're outside your comfort zone—and especially when you feel like you "can't." Every time you push yourself further into the discomfort, you redefine your limits and become stronger and more resilient. And you feel great for it. It works the same way when you endeavor in the opposite direction while doing restorative yoga.

Once again, how you are on the mat is a mirror of how you are everywhere. If you can't deal with the discomfort that might accompany the unfamiliar sensation of lengthening the front of your body when you're relaxing on the floor, how are you going to handle the exhaustion that accompanies the last few miles of your marathon?

In the process of being present with what's happening on the mat, restorative yoga helps you to more clearly discern between tension and relaxation, increases self-awareness, and builds the mental and emotional strength required to best manage whatever comes at you. Even more important, it deepens your connection to the only person responsible for achieving your goals: you.

LET GO

Letting go is easier said than done. And resistance to releasing stress, tension, and emotion is usually a habit, not a choice. Adding context—becoming clear about where negative holding patterns exist, and why—will help you melt resistance.

Even when you give yourself permission to relax, your body might continue to hold on. This is why recovery and rest days don't necessarily go hand in hand. When left unchecked, physical tension is like a prop that helps to hold us up to meet challenges and then is difficult to remove when it's no longer needed. That's because without regular, intentional practice, it's easy to forget how to let go.

The PNS can be the trigger for letting go, and restorative yoga helps you to pull that trigger.

LETTING GO = Releasing physical, mental, and emotional tension

Let go a little bit right now:

- Stop what you're doing and acknowledge that you're pausing to ease tension so that you can feel more relaxed.

- Scan your body and notice where the tension is—especially in common tension spots like your jaw, forehead, shoulders, and abdomen.

- See if you can simply use your heightened awareness of where tension is living in your body to begin to soften those spots.

- Now relax them even more.

- Continue to let go.

GET REAL

What am I holding on to that's
impeding my pursuit of my goals?

What's stopping me
from letting go right now?

When I let go I feel:

How to Do Restorative Yoga

There are two ways to use restorative yoga to work in:

RELAX DEEPLY

Static (still) postures, many of which make use of props,
to open the body and encourage deep physical and mental relaxation.

GENTLY MOBILIZE

Small movements that increase fluidity to muscles, surrounding tissues,
and joints to ease stiffness and restore range of motion.

HOW TO REST YOUR SPINE IN NEUTRAL

To help relax your back, be sure to rest your spine in neutral whenever possible—especially when lying on your back. Even in poses where you are twisting or side bending or applying mobility, increasing your awareness of your spinal alignment will help you bring more ease to this area.

➲ Sit or lie down and set up for whatever posture you're about to do.

➲ Arch and round your back a few times (similar to cat/cow pose in yoga) to feel all available alignments.

➲ Stop in the middle—the midpoint between the two extremes of arching and rounding—and keep your spine there.

➲ Now put both of your hands onto your waist and make sure you have an even amount of space between your ribs and hips on both your right and left side.

➲ Aim to maintain this neutral position whenever possible.

HOW TO GET STARTED

WHEN: For recovery purposes, it's ideal to use these practices post-workout or as you wind down your day.

WHAT: Choose a pose or routine based on how you feel and how much time you have available. Because you will hold the poses for a longer duration, expect to do a few poses rather than a bunch (unless you really have a lot of time to spend). For example, in a 10-minute session you might do two postures, or in 30 minutes you might do five.

DURATION: Like meditation, longer is better. The longer you hold a pose, the more time your body has to settle in, unwind, and relax deeply, allowing you to target specific muscles and areas of the body while also calming your nervous system. Aim for a minimum of 5 minutes per posture and up to 15 minutes.

WHERE: A quiet, unrushed, relaxing setting is ideal. That being said, for recovery to fit into your life, it has to be practical. You can still enhance your recovery with some restorative poses while loud music plays at your gym, or on the floor of your living room, or in the moments just before you jump into the shower—as long as you give working in your full attention.

BREATHE: Default to inhaling and exhaling through your nose, unless you pair your pose with a breath-focused meditation that suggests a different technique.

PROP YOURSELF

Traditional restorative yoga asks you to support yourself with many props and hold postures for a long time, which feels amazing and has many benefits. But for the sake of practicality and accessibility, the restorative poses in this book are shorter in duration and rely on fewer props—mostly items that you already have around your home. No yoga bolster? No big deal.

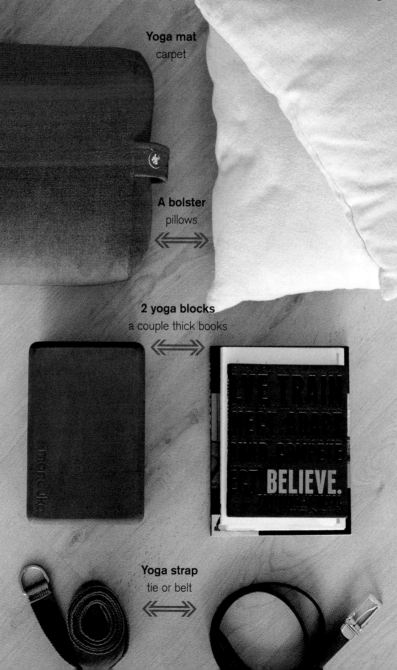

Yoga mat
carpet

A bolster
pillows

2 yoga blocks
a couple thick books

BELIEVE.

Yoga strap
tie or belt

WORK IN
FOR PHYSICAL RELAXATION

Use these simple postures, movements, and routines to help you incorporate yoga into your training, try different techniques, and ultimately make it a real—practical—part of your recovery routine.

These postures are organized by deep relaxation and gentle mobility. See the pose notes for more on specific areas of the body impacted plus additional benefits. Pick a couple of poses (or just one!) based on the time you have available, using the pose notes to select what's most appropriate based on how your body feels. For example, if you've been hunched over the handlebars on your bike for hours, mobilizing your shoulders and upper back will help to increase circulation to the areas that are static when you ride, greatly aiding the recovery process in a way that directly addresses what you've just done. Or, if you have more time available, use one of the specific routines suggested at the end of this chapter (pp. 154–157). As you become familiar with all these tools, it will become easy to select postures that are relevant to your body.

GAME PLAN

⇒ Select a pose or routine and get comfortable.

⇒ Pause and notice how you feel; use the pre-/post-game (p. 94).

⇒ Set a timer for however long you plan to spend in the posture, or go by feel
and stay until you're ready to move on or end your practice.

⇒ When the timer ends or you are finished, pause and feel the difference;
use the pre-/post-game again.

⇒ Onward!

Refer to **THE PLAN: RECOVER FOR REAL** (p. 162) for a month-long plan for more inspiration on how to get started.

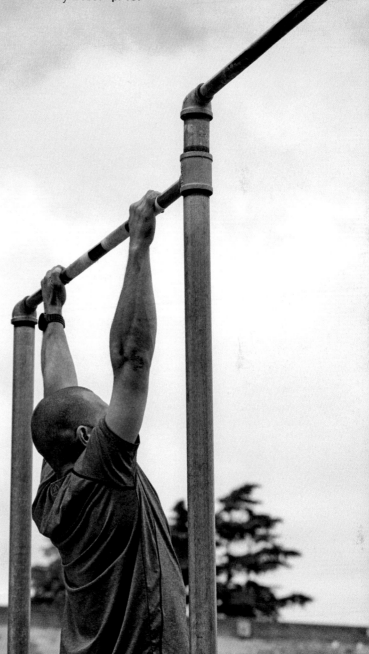

HOW TO ALIGN YOUR NECK

Especially during recovery, head placement and accompanying neck alignment matters. There is a nerve in your neck that significantly impacts your nervous system. The vagus nerve is the longest of your cranial nerves and passes through your neck all the way down into your abdomen. When not aligned optimally, it can impede your PNS from doing its thing: It can stifle your relaxation response.

Typical posture today, largely the result of the amount of sitting we do, has your head coming forward more than it should and creating excess strain. Your head is heavy so it's no surprise that your neck isn't happy when you move it beyond its intended alignment over your shoulders. When you take that posture to the floor and lie down on your back, you will find that you are looking up and slightly back because your neck is overextended, leaving your chin higher than your forehead. It's not only uncomfortable—it puts a damper on your restorative mojo.

SITTING TALL. You can remedy this alignment problem to optimize relaxation in meditation and seated postures by focusing on lengthening the back of your neck and imagining you're trying to give yourself a double chin as you move your head back in space.

YES

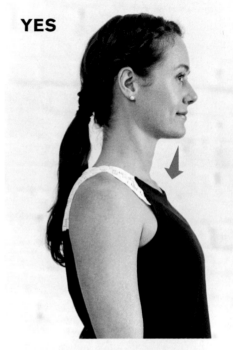

NO

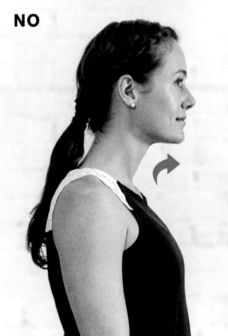

LYING DOWN. Become more aware of this common misalignment by leaning a mirror or your phone camera against a wall next to you when you lie down so you can see for yourself, or ask someone to check for you.

⇢ Your chin and forehead should be level.

⇢ If your chin is higher than your forehead and you can't find neutral simply by lengthening the back of your neck, place a small folded towel beneath the back of your head to level things off and ease any tension in your neck and throat.

YES

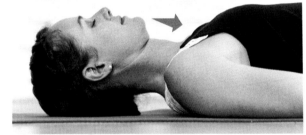

NO

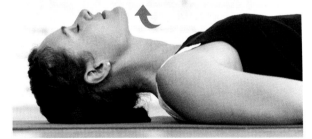

HOW DOES YOUR BODY FEEL?

BEFORE YOU PRACTICE: Pause and notice how you feel. These observations give you a baseline for comparison when you are finished, help you to feel the difference, and carry the benefits forward.

⇒ How does your body feel?

⇒ Are there any specific areas of tension or stiffness in your body? Where?

⇒ What do the sensations in those areas feel like? Be specific.

AFTER YOU PRACTICE: Pause and feel the difference. Use the same questions to check in post-yoga. Taking this extra moment helps you become aware of the effects of your practice, absorb the benefits, and feel motivated to continue.

Pause and *feel the difference.*

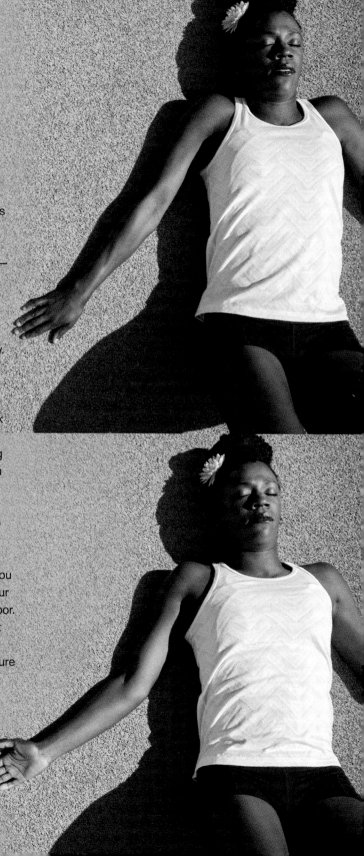

PALMS UP

Most people naturally turn their palms toward the floor when they lie down. Whether you realize it or not, this mirrors common postural imbalance—due to heavy training and lots of sitting—that stiffens the chest and internally rotates (turns in) the upper arm bones. When the palms face back, you may hunch forward slightly.

Instead, rotate your upper arm bones so your palms face up or forward, which opens the chest and helps the shoulder blades move back and down.

If your chest is tight from training and sitting, you may notice that when you try to do this, the backs of your hands don't easily touch the floor. When left suspended with nothing to rest on, this places excess strain on your shoulders. So it's important that when you turn your palms forward, you find an arm placement that allows your knuckles to rest heavily against the floor.

Practice making this your default any time you lie down, which will ultimately help you improve your posture when you're standing.

Try it now!

CHILD'S POSE

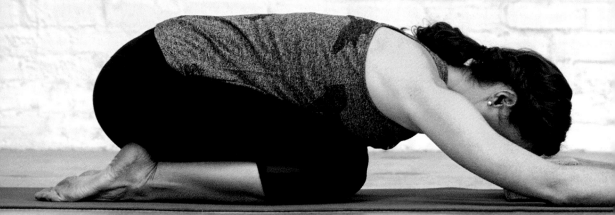

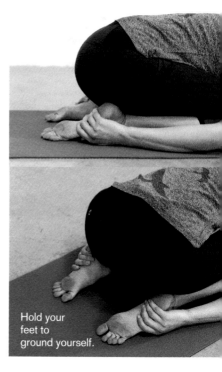

Hold your feet to ground yourself.

WHY

Eases shoulder, back, and hip stiffness.

HOW

Kneel with your legs hip-width apart, keeping your shins parallel.

Lengthen your torso down onto your thighs.

Reach your arms forward, palms down, or rest them back along your sides, palms up.

Rest your forehead on the floor or a block.

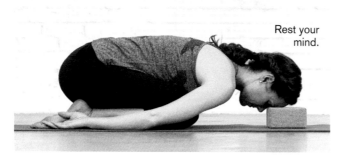

Rest your mind.

TIP: *If your neck is uncomfortable, place a block underneath your forehead to help neutralize it.*

WHY

A bolster or pillow facilitates deeper relaxation while easing shoulder, back, and hip stiffness.

HOW

Kneel with your legs wider than hip-width apart and pull a bolster between your legs, keeping your shins parallel.

Lengthen your torso down onto the bolster—if it feels too far for your torso to reach, add additional props to increase its height.

Rest your arms forward alongside the bolster, palms down.

Turn your head to one side.

Halfway through the time you are spending here, turn your head in the other direction.

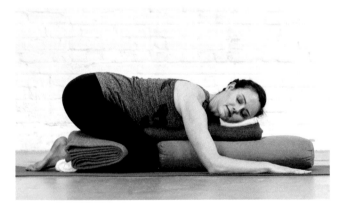

TIP: *If your feet are uncomfortable, place a blanket or towel roll beneath your ankles; if your knees are uncomfortable, place extra padding between your calves and hamstrings— helping to create more space for tender areas.*

SUPPORTED CHILD'S POSE

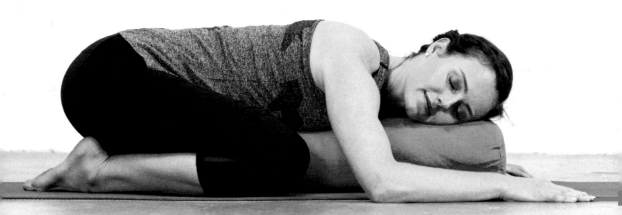

Relax the front of your body
into the support beneath you.

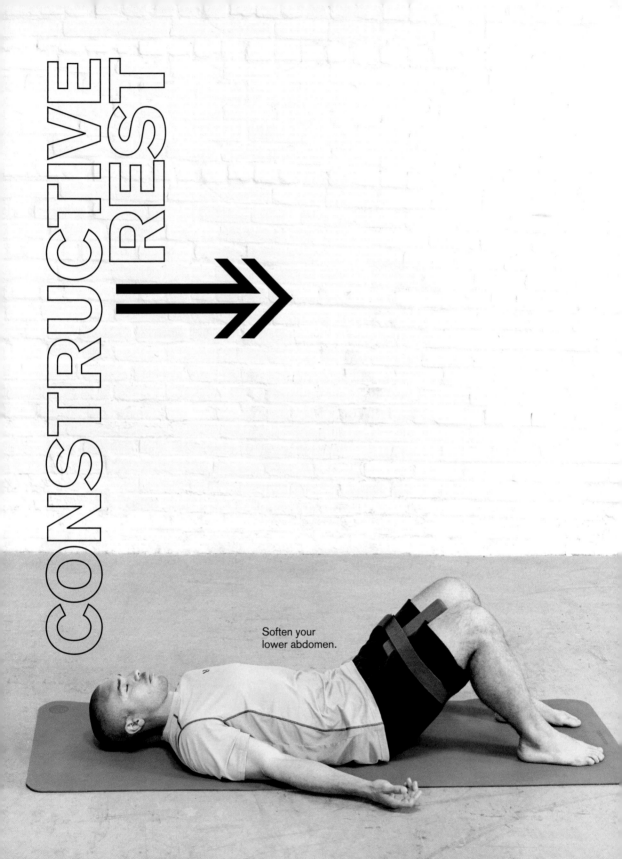

CONSTRUCTIVE REST ⟹

Soften your
lower abdomen.

WHY

Encourages the tops of the thigh bones to drop back and down, relaxing the lower abdominals and back, and, most noticeably, the psoas—a powerful hip flexor.

HOW

Put a block lengthwise between your thighs and loop a strap around your thighs (it should be tight!).

Lie on your back with your knees bent, feet parallel on the floor.

Rest your arms open, palms up.

WHY

Relaxes the hips and low back.

HOW

Lie on your back and rest your arms open, palms up.

Bring your feet wider than hip-width (about as wide as your mat if you're using one) and drop your thighs together into a triangle shape.

TRY IT

FOCUS ON CONTACT WITH THE FLOOR

Especially if you are feeling anxious, it's helpful to focus on the places where your body is in contact with the floor, which gives you a focal point to help ground and calm your mind.

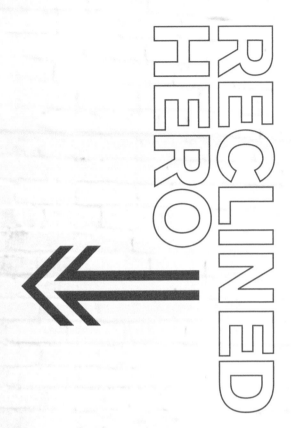

RECLINED HERO

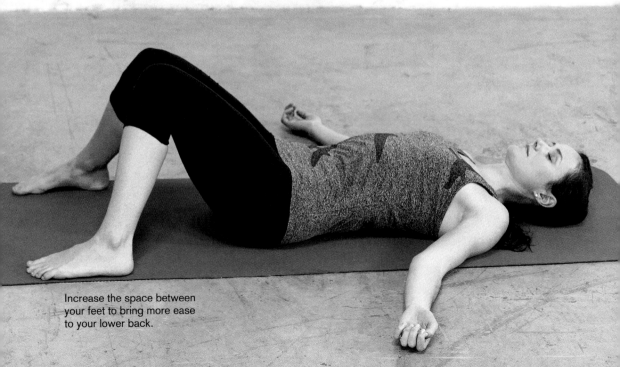

Increase the space between your feet to bring more ease to your lower back.

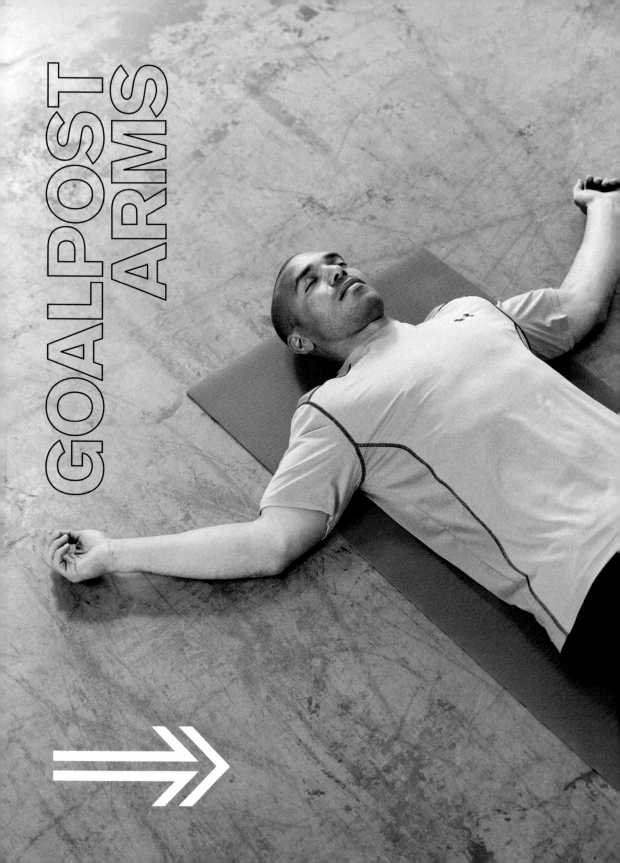

GOALPOST ARMS

WHY

Opens the chest.

HOW

Lie on your back.

Bend your arms into a goalpost shape so that your elbows are bent slightly wider than 90 degrees, palms up.

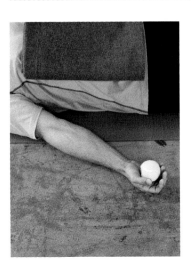

TRY IT

ADD WEIGHT

When resting in restorative postures, it can help to add weight to various points on your body. This causes those places to feel heavier and can help you feel more grounded and supported, encouraging deeper relaxation. For example, try gently holding tennis balls in your hands, allowing your fingers to relax around them, or place a folded blanket on your abdomen.

WHY

Relaxes the back.

HOW

Place a bolster under your knees lengthwise and turn your thighs out so that your feet turn away from each other slightly.

Lie on your back.

Rest your arms open, palms up.

TIP: If your low back is arched, lie over a folded blanket so that your rib cage is on the blanket.

TRY IT

ADJUST AS NEEDED

It's kind of like the fairy tale *The Princess and the Pea*—you can't relax if there's anything bothering your nervous system. It's worth it to keep adjusting until you're absolutely sure you're comfortable. Then, when you're settled, acknowledge that you're settled. This will also help you more deliberately relax.

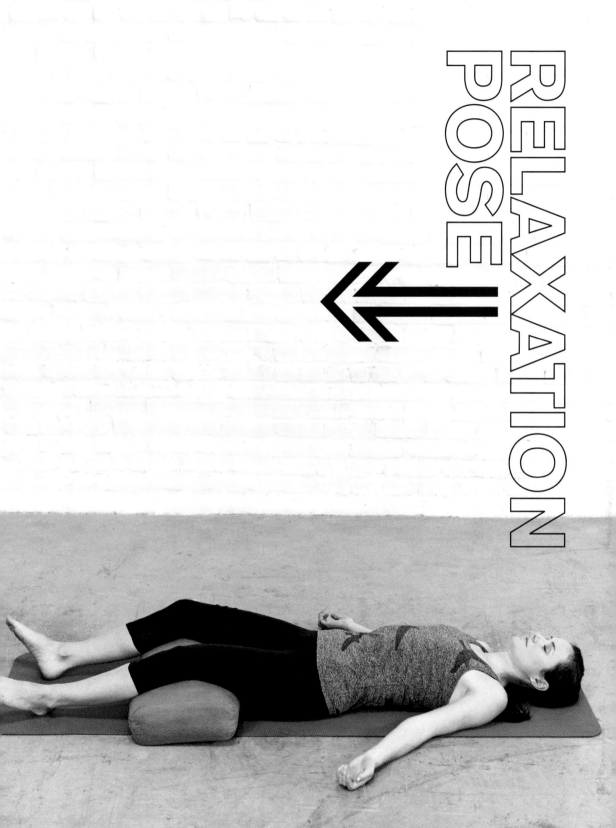

RELAXATION POSE

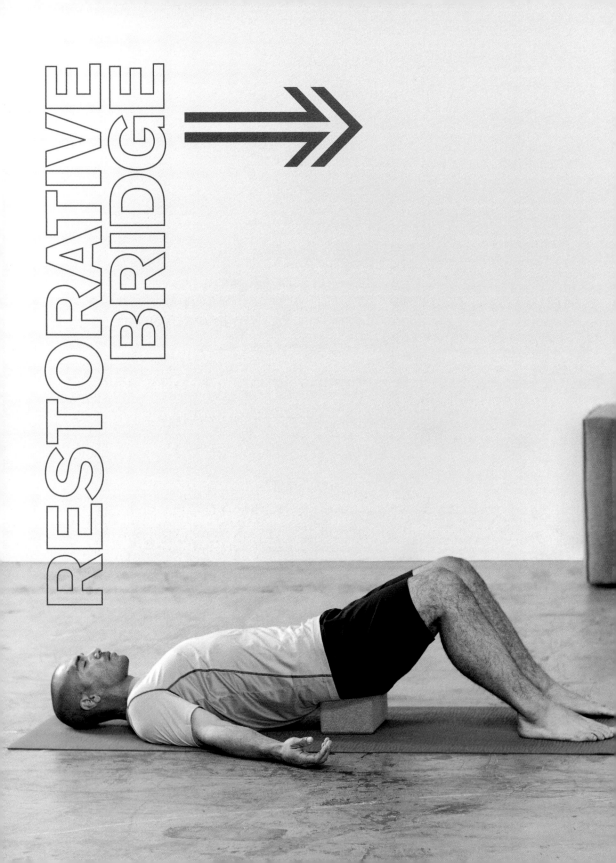

RESTORATIVE BRIDGE →

WHY

Increases circulation, lengthens the front body (especially the hips and the shoulders), and helps to neutralize the spine.

HOW

Lie on your back with your knees bent, feet parallel on the floor.

Put a block (or other prop, approximately 6 inches thick) under your low back—don't let your butt hang forward off the block.

Rest your arms open, palms up.

WHY

Stretches and increases circulation in side-body connective tissue.

HOW

Sit and pull a bolster horizontally against your hip.

Lie over the bolster so that it lifts and lengthens the space between your ribs and hips on both sides of your body.

Stack your legs and bend your knees slightly, resting your top foot into the sole of your bottom foot.

Rest your head on your bottom arm, and reach your top arm overhead.

Repeat on the other side.

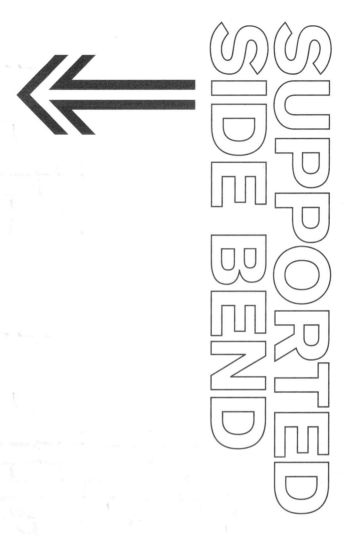

SUPPORTED SIDE BEND

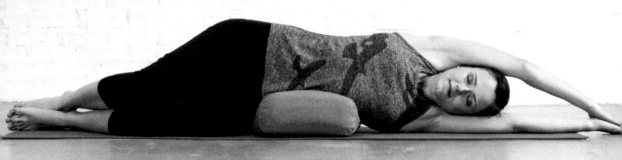

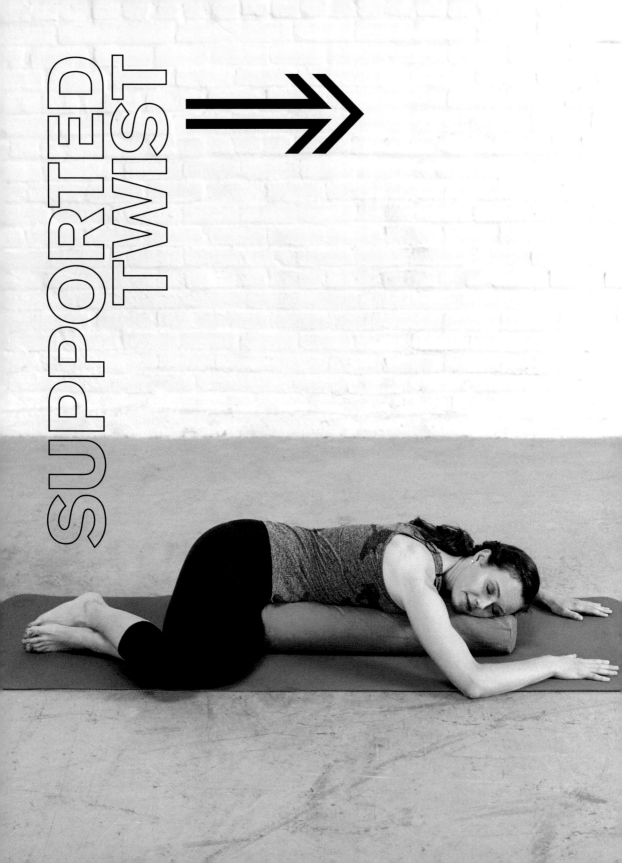

SUPPORTED TWIST →→

WHY

Relaxes the back.

HOW

Sit down with your legs staggered, resting your top foot into the sole of your bottom foot.

Pull a bolster against the side of your upper thigh.

Turn toward your prop and lengthen your torso down onto it.

Rest your arms in a goalpost shape, palms down.

Turn your head in the opposite direction as your legs if it's comfortable, if not, keep your head turned in the same direction as your legs.

Repeat on the other side.

TIP: If your knees are uncomfortable, place extra padding between your thighs.

TRY IT

LENGTHEN, DON'T FLOP

You get to lie face-down in many restorative postures, promoting spinal length—which in turn supports optimal posture. This also adds support for the front of your body, which is incredibly calming for your nervous system. As you set up, be sure to lengthen your spine as much as you can and maintain as much of that length as possible as you lie on your prop.

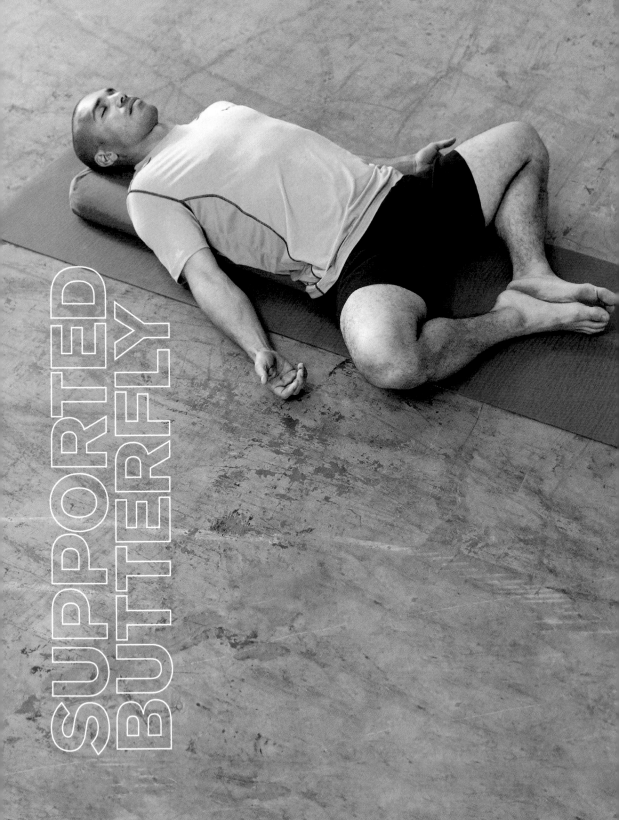

SUPPORTED BUTTERFLY

WHY

Opens the chest and hips.

HOW

Sit down, pull a bolster lengthwise against your butt, and bring the soles of your feet together.

Lie back over the prop, keeping your butt on the floor.

Rest your arms open, palms up.

TIP: If your knees are uncomfortable, support them by placing props beneath your thighs.

SUPPORTED BRIDGE

→→

Feel the front of your
body lift and open.

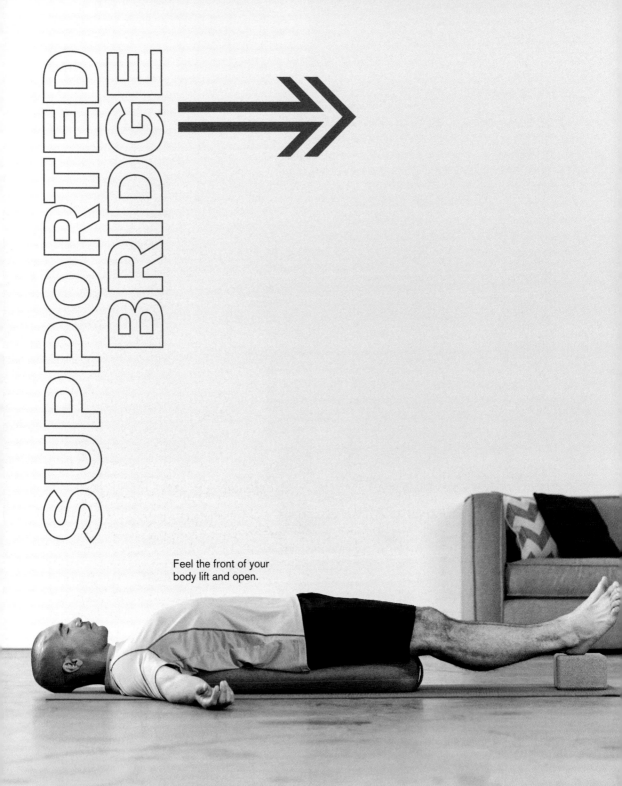

WHY

Opens the front of the body.

HOW

Put a block a few feet in front of a lengthwise bolster on the floor.

Sit on the middle of the bolster and lie back over it so that your upper back, arms, and head are on the floor.

Put your feet on top of the block and turn your thighs out so that your feet turn away from each other slightly.

Rest your arms open, palms up.

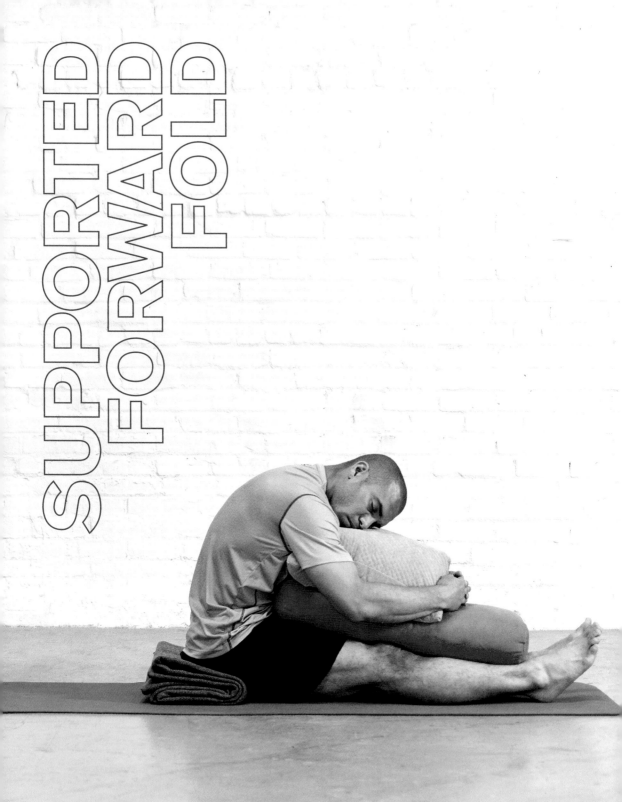

SUPPORTED FORWARD FOLD

WHY

Stretches and increases circulation in hamstrings and back-body connective tissue.

HOW

Sit on the edge of a folded blanket with a bolster extended lengthwise on your legs.

Lengthen your torso down onto your bolster—add as much height as needed to the stack so that it's easy for your torso to reach.

Rest your arms forward, palms down.

Turn your head to one side.

Halfway through the time you are spending here, turn your head in the other direction.

WHY

Eases back and abdominal tension, relaxes the front of the body.

HOW

Place a folded blanket horizontally about six inches wide and no higher than three inches tall on the floor in front of you.

Lengthen down onto the blanket so that it spans the area between your ribs and hips—your hip bones should be on the floor.

Stack your palms and rest your forehead on top.

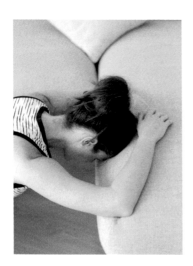

TRY IT

REST YOUR FOREHEAD

Mental strain and accompanying facial tension can be stubborn because they're such deeply ingrained habits. A simple way to address this in forward-lying restorative postures is to release the work of holding your head by adding support for your forehead, helping to calm peripheral nerves, which is incredibly calming for your nervous system.

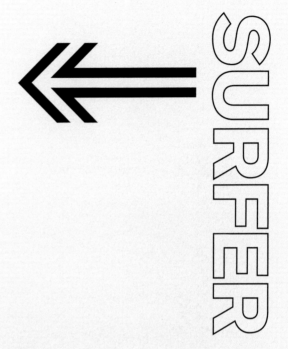

SURFER

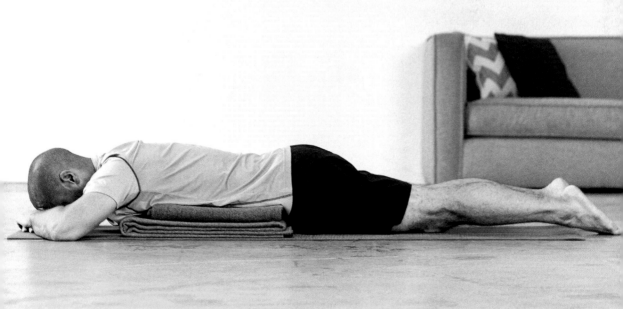

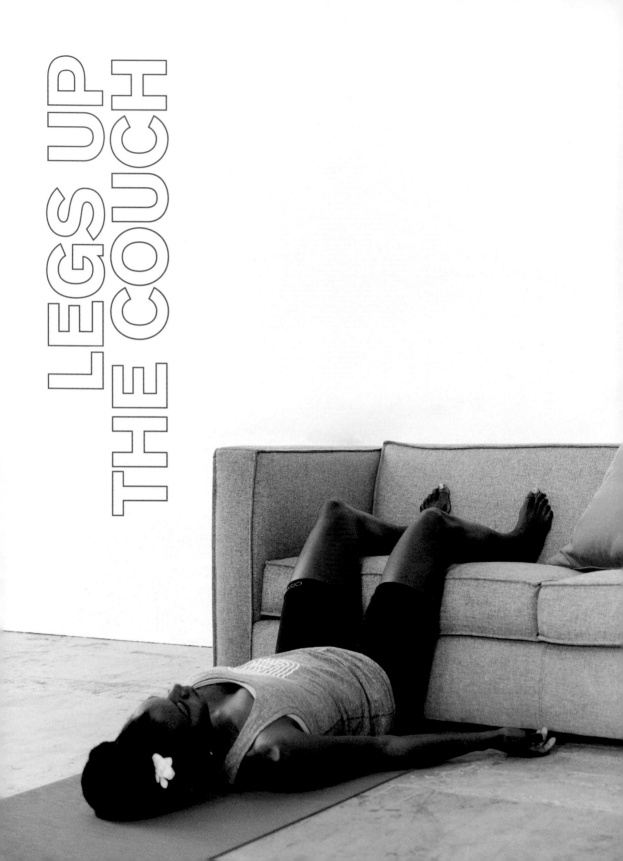

LEGS UP
THE COUCH

WHY

Relaxes the back, recirculates excess blood and fluid in the legs.

HOW

Lie down on the floor, bend your knees, and rest your lower legs on a couch, chair, or ottoman.

Rest your arms open, palms up.

TRY IT

KEEP GOING

When you think you're relaxed, don't stop. Keep going into it. Just like you keep pushing to redefine your boundaries when you work out, keep going when you work in. When you think you're relaxed, you can probably relax even more. Stay with it.

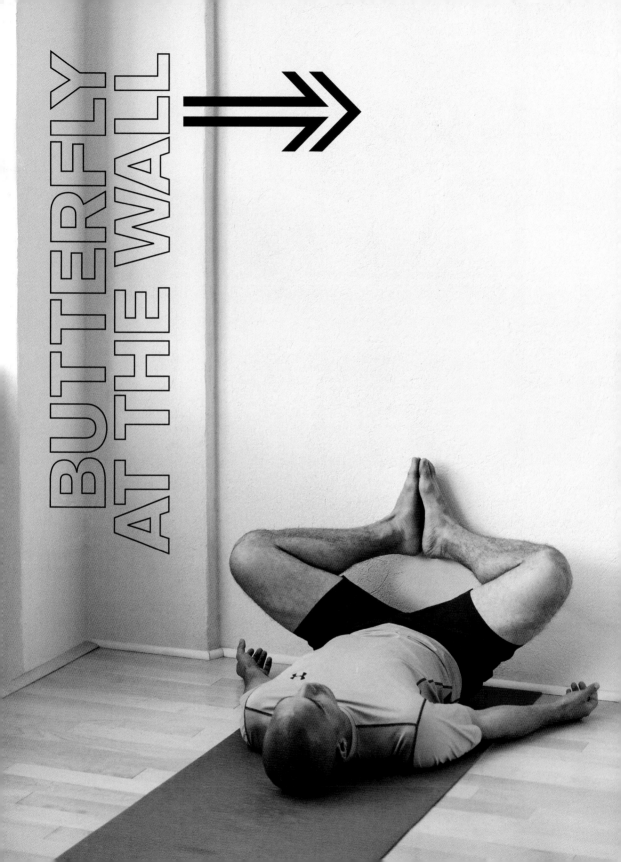

BUTTERFLY AT THE WALL →

WHY

Opens the hips and recirculates excess blood and fluid in the legs.

HOW

Lie on your back and put your legs up the wall, moving as far back as needed to neutralize your spine.

Bring the soles of your feet together so that your feet and all your toes connect—if your knees, hips, or back are uncomfortable, move farther away from the wall.

Rest your arms open, palms up.

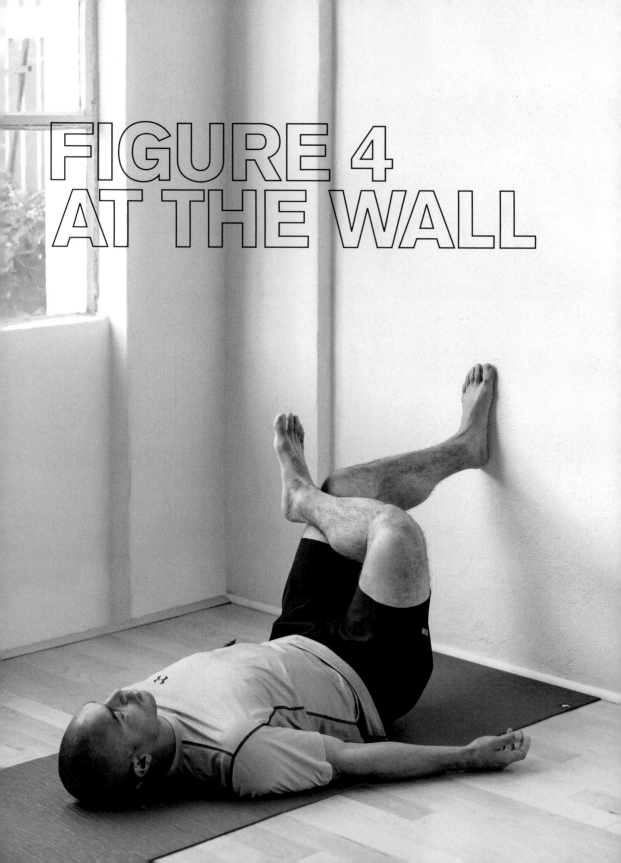

FIGURE 4
AT THE WALL

WHY

Opens the hips, relaxes the back, and recirculates excess blood and fluid in the legs.

HOW

Lie on your back and put your feet flat on the wall so that your knees are bent at about a 90-degree angle—if your knees, hips, or back are uncomfortable, move farther away from the wall.

Cross one ankle over your other knee, keeping that foot flexed, and keeping the knee of the leg that is touching the wall aligned over the ankle.

If needed, slide your foot farther up the wall to get the ankle crossed over the knee while keeping your spine neutral.

Rest your arms open, palms up.

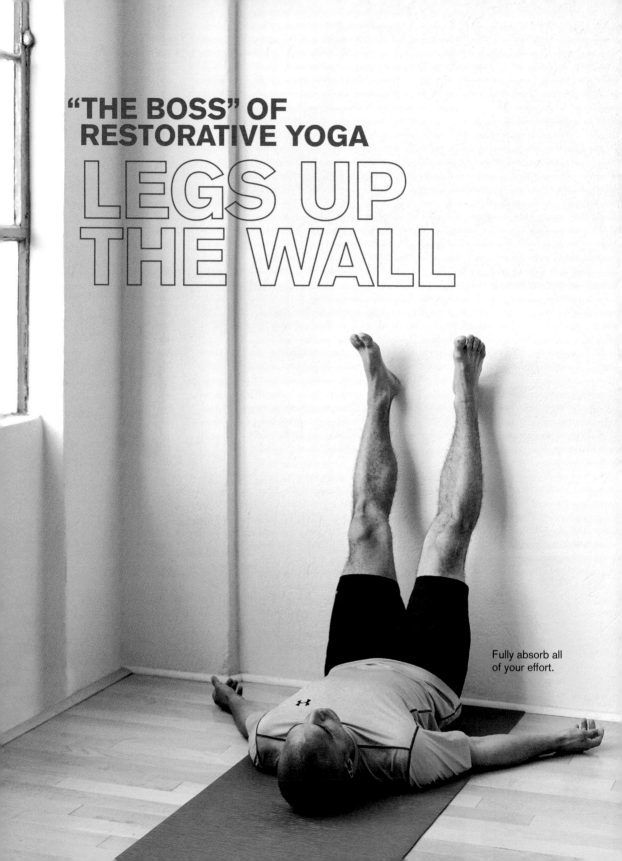

"THE BOSS" OF RESTORATIVE YOGA

LEGS UP THE WALL

Fully absorb all of your effort.

WHY

Recirculates the blood and any excess fluid in the legs, opens the hamstrings, relaxes the low back and feet, and more.

HOW

Lie on your back and extend your legs up the wall, moving as far back as needed to neutralize your spine.

Bend your knees slightly and turn your feet away from each other.

Rest your arms open, palms up.

TIP: For an added recovery boost, put a bolster under your butt and loop a strap around your calves, creating additional support for your body to rest into.

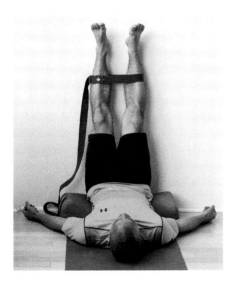

NECK CIRCLES

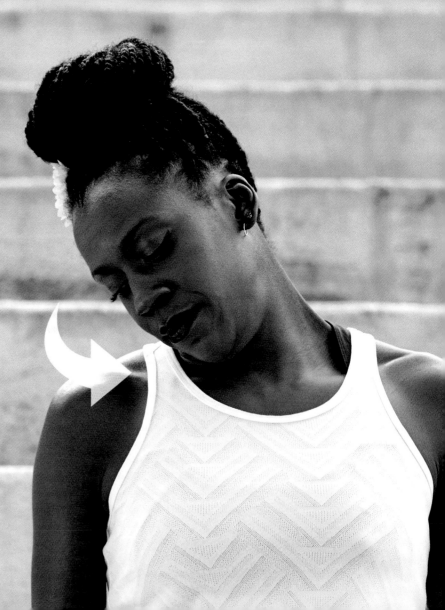

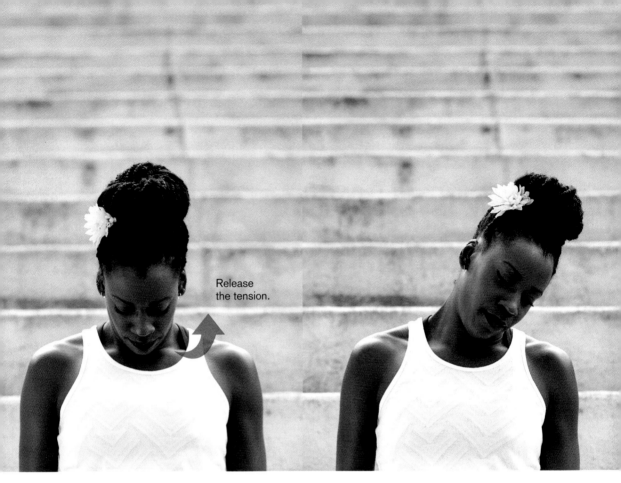

Release
the tension.

HOW

Sit comfortably.

Drop your chin toward your chest.

Circle your head to one shoulder.

Drop your head back down to center, then circle it to the other shoulder.

Continue for about 10 reps.

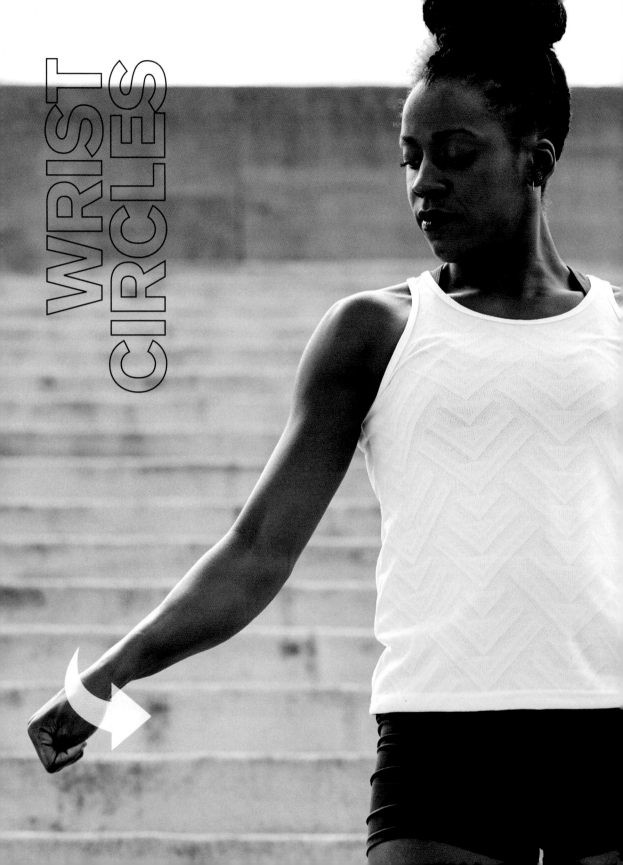

WRIST CIRCLES

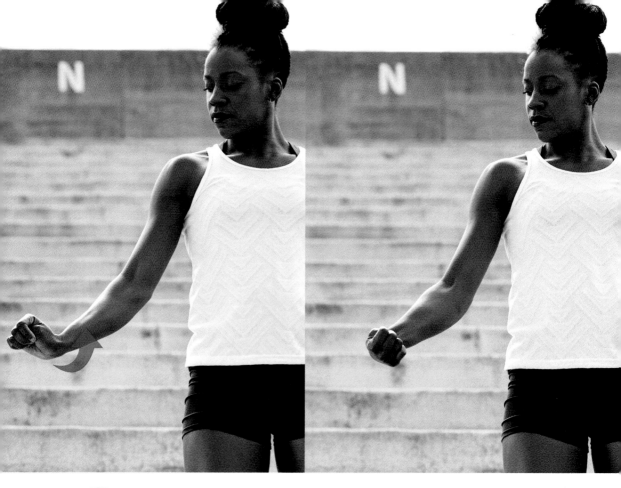

HOW

Stand or sit comfortably.

Bring your thumbs into the palms of your hands and wrap the rest of your fingers around them, creating fists.

Circle your wrists 5–10 times in each direction.

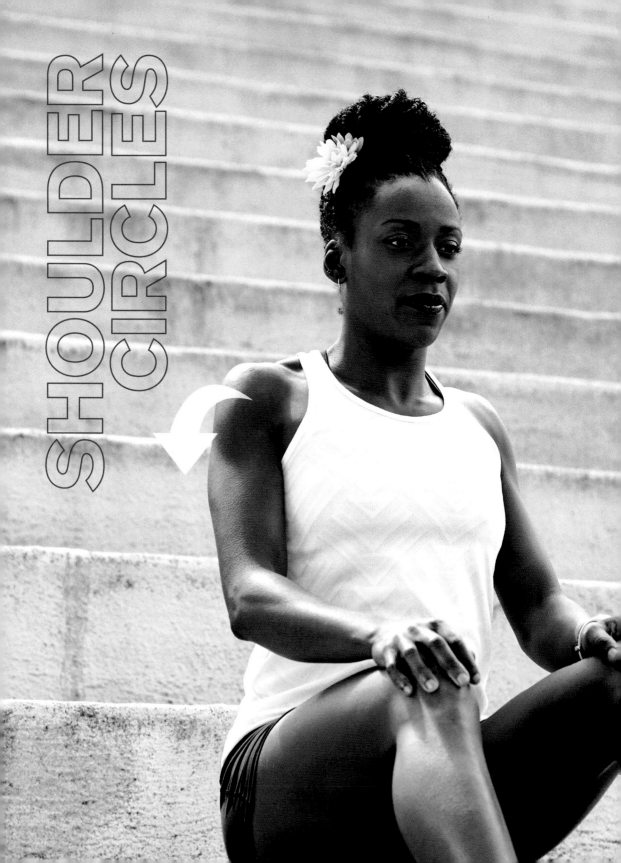

SHOULDER CIRCLES

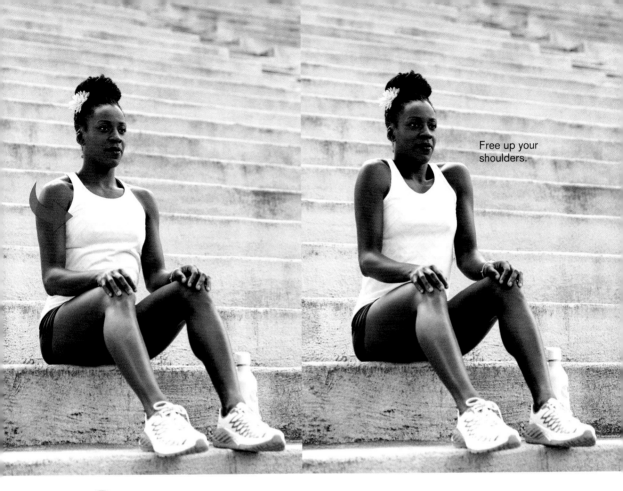

Free up your
shoulders.

HOW

Sit comfortably or come onto all fours (see pp. 136–137).

Circle your shoulders.

Do 5–10 circles in each direction.

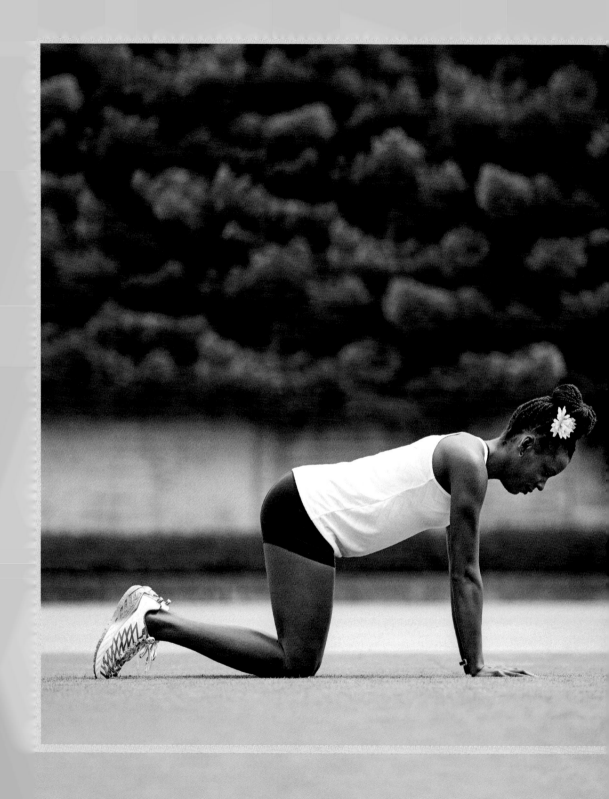

HOW TO ALIGN ON ALL FOURS

Being on your hands and knees is the starting point for many yoga poses, so set yourself up for success by initiating a solid foundation to work from. Keep in mind also that your knees aren't well designed for bearing weight—when you come onto all fours you can feel how they have no natural padding; it's basically bone against surface. Keep them comfortable and safe by putting a folded blanket or towel beneath them, especially if you're not practicing on a soft surface.

- ⇗ Come onto all fours.

- ⇗ Place your legs hip-width apart with your knees under your hips and your shins parallel.

- ⇗ Place your hands under your shoulders without locking your elbows, and spread your fingers wide.

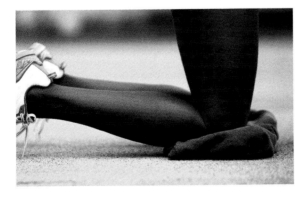

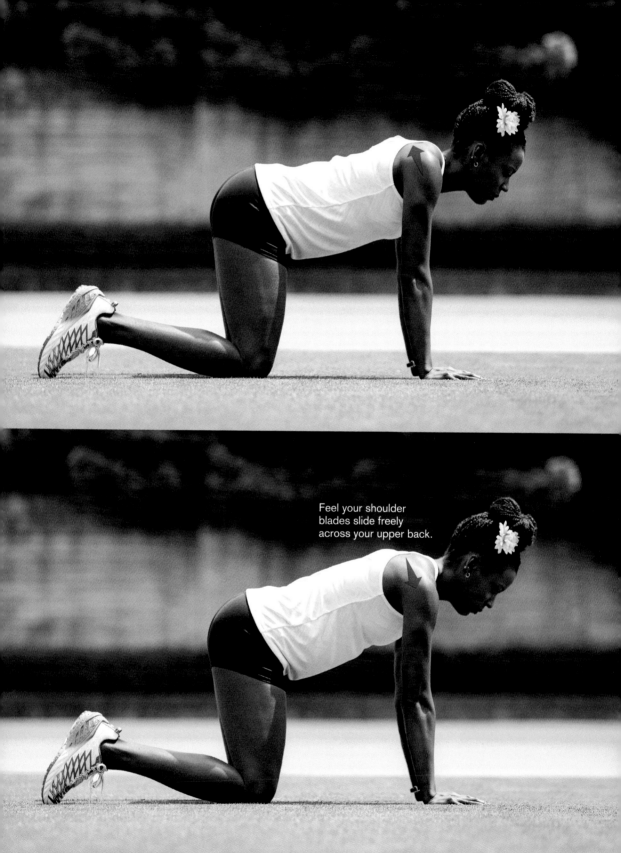

Feel your shoulder
blades slide freely
across your upper back.

SHOULDER ROW

HOW

Come onto all fours and drop your chest between your shoulders, feeling your shoulder blades move closer together.

Round your upper back, feeling your shoulder blades move farther apart.

Continue for 10 reps.

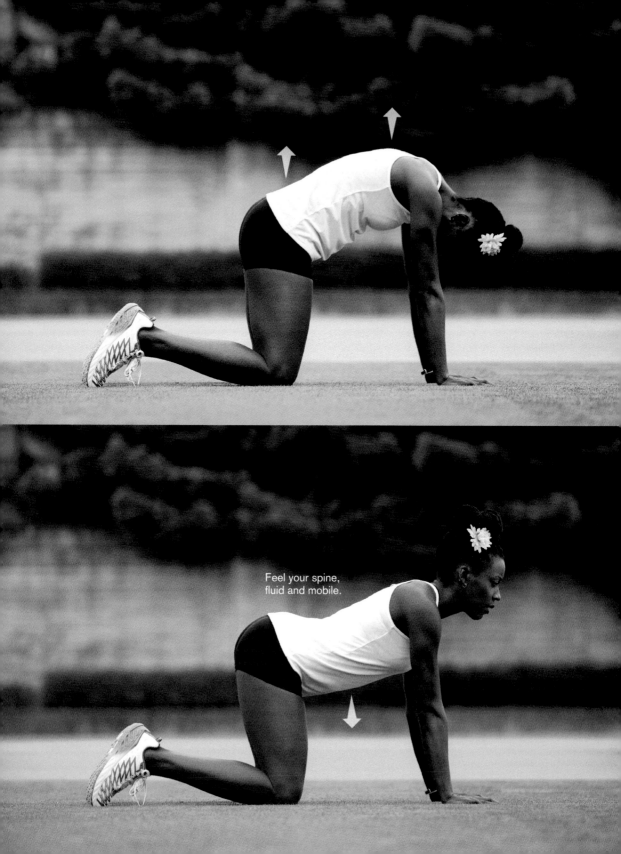

Feel your spine,
fluid and mobile.

CAT/COW

HOW

Come onto all fours.

Round your spine and take your chin toward your chest, dropping your head.

Lift your hips, chest, and chin and drop your abdomen toward the floor.

Continue for 10 reps.

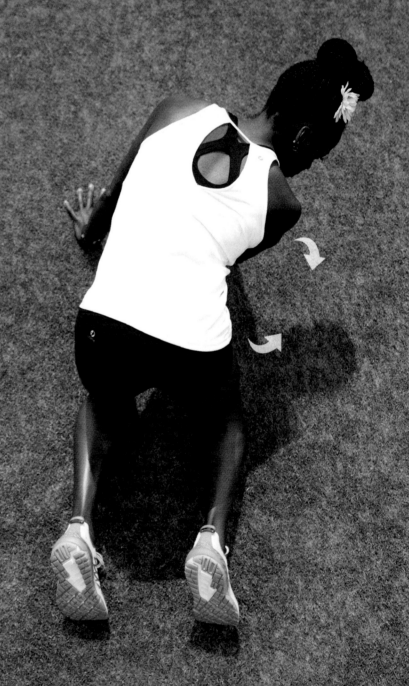

ALL FOURS
SIDE BEND

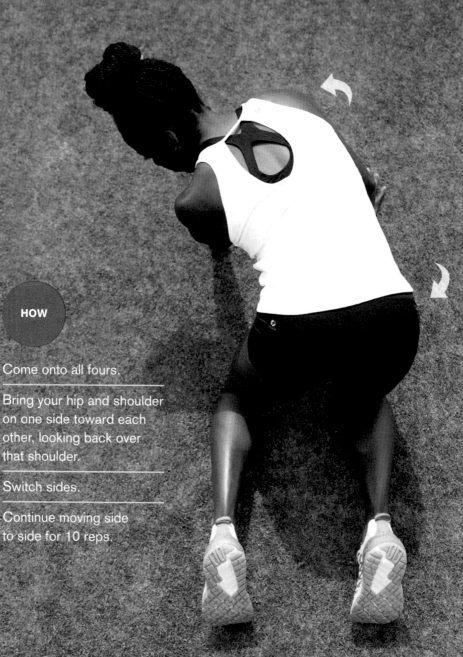

HOW

Come onto all fours.

Bring your hip and shoulder on one side toward each other, looking back over that shoulder.

Switch sides.

Continue moving side to side for 10 reps.

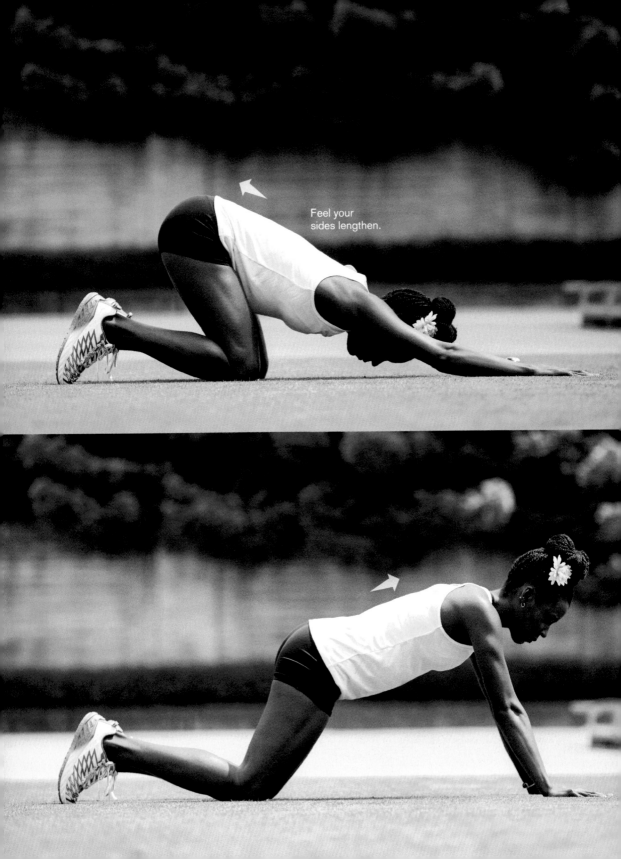

Feel your
sides lengthen.

FORWARD/ BACK

HOW

Come onto all fours and move your knees a few inches back from your hips
(as if you were moving toward a knees-down push-up position).

Rock your weight back as far as you can.

Rock your weight forward, returning to where you started.

Continue for 10 reps.

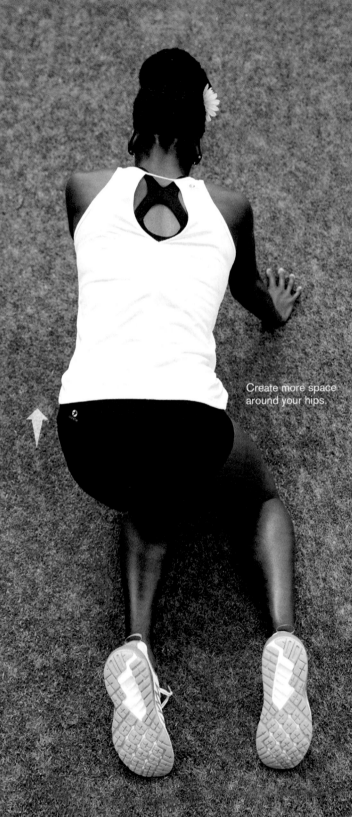

HIP ROCKING

Create more space around your hips.

Come onto all fours.

Lean your hips to one side and keep them there as you rock forward and back 5–10 times, then switch sides.

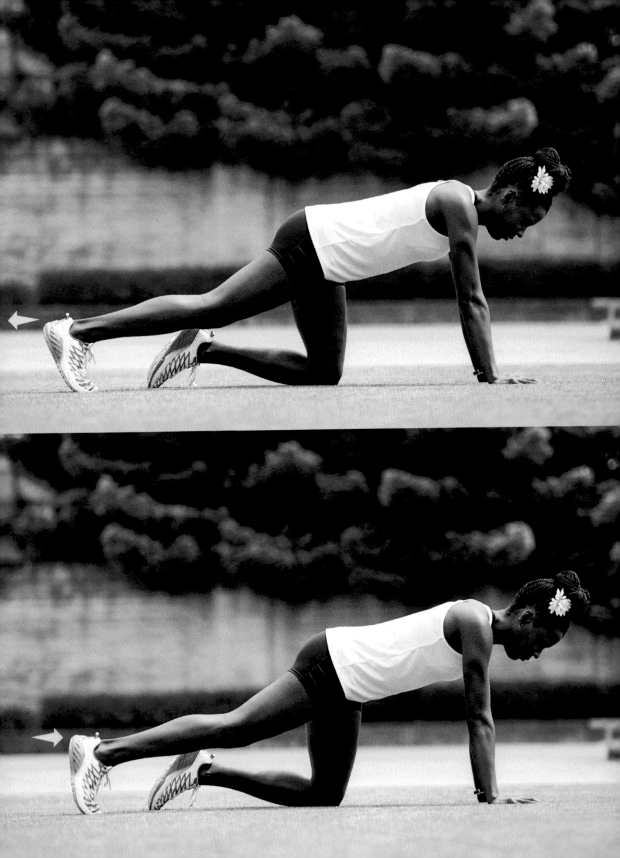

CALF PUMP

HOW

Come onto all fours.

Straighten one leg behind you, tucking your toes under on the floor.

Keeping your hips level, rock forward and back, as if you're doing standing heel lifts on that leg.

Continue for 10 reps, then switch sides.

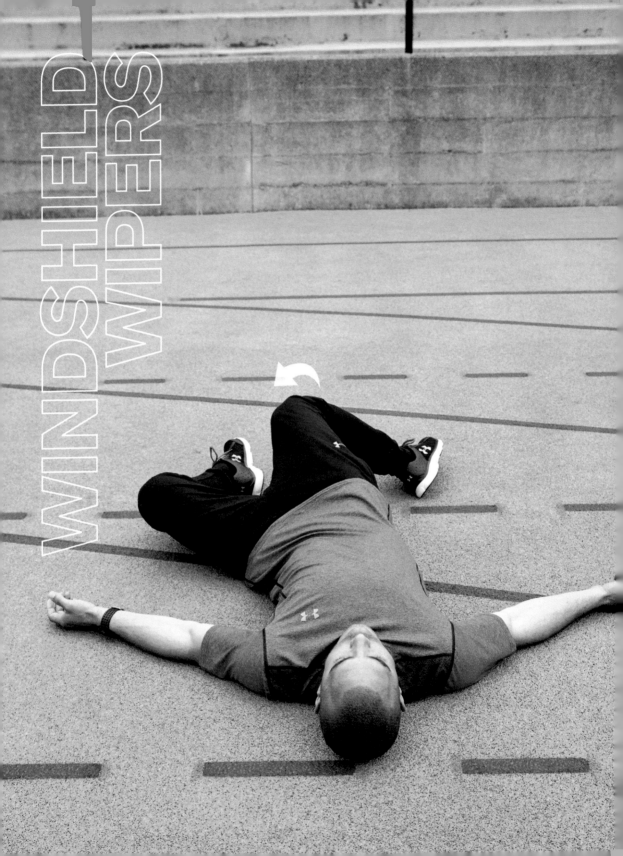

WINDSHIELD WIPERS

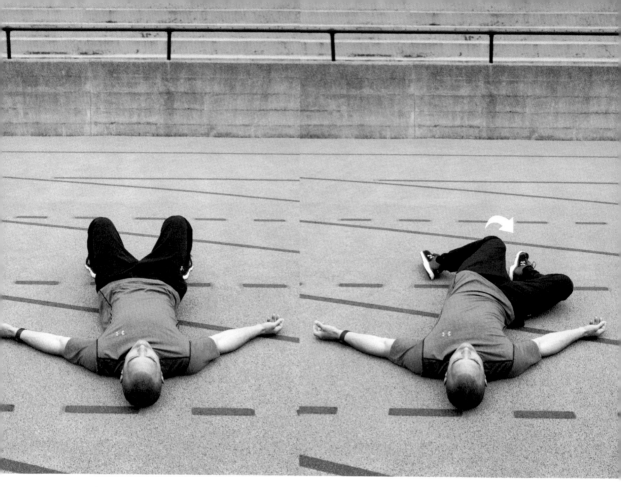

HOW

Sit or lie down with your knees bent and your feet wider than hip-width (about as wide as your mat if you're using one).

Rest your arms open, palms up.

Drop your knees to one side.

Lift your knees back to center, then drop them to the other side.

Continue for about 20 reps.

EASE HEAD, FACE & NECK TENSION

Most people unconsciously hold a lot of tension in their face and neck—especially the throat, jaw, the space between the eyebrows, and skin on the forehead. These spots are often home to activated trigger points, which are bundles of fascia (like connective tissue) and/or muscle that can refer pain patterns to regions elsewhere along their fascia but not always necessarily to the specific point itself. This is what distinguishes them from tender spots. These trigger points significantly impact areas like the neck, eyes, shoulders, jaw, and chest, and are a major contributor to headaches. Because these areas are also situated closest to your brain, as tension builds they can take over your concentration and drain your energy—even if you're not aware of it.

While you can become aware of tension and work on consciously relaxing these spots, applying direct pressure to those tender trigger points can significantly relieve many forms of head, face, and neck tension. Bringing more ease to related muscles can help you feel more clear and focused, resulting in a noticeable reduction in your perception of stress. Try this self-massage now or the next time you're in a restorative yoga posture.

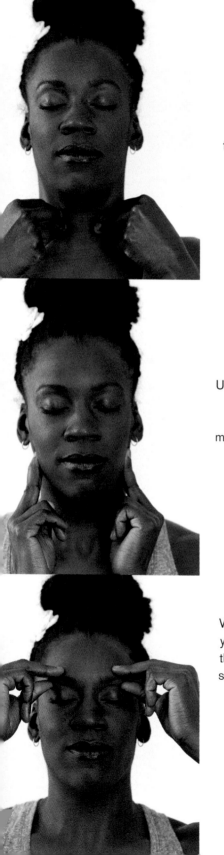

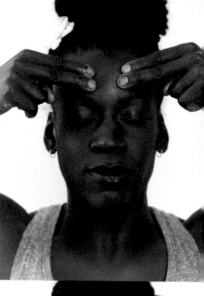

1

With your thumbs and the side of your index fingers closest to your thumbs, gently pinch the thin but prominent muscles of your neck that run diagonally from your skull to clavicle—move up and down the neck a couple times as you do this.

2

Use your fingertips to massage your jaw in a circular motion for about 30 seconds.

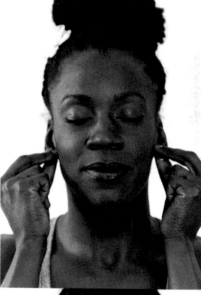

3

Use your thumbs and index fingers to gently pinch your eyebrows, beginning in the middle and moving to the ends a couple times.

4

Use a few fingertips to gently press in the center of your forehead, and then stroke horizontally to your hairline a few times.

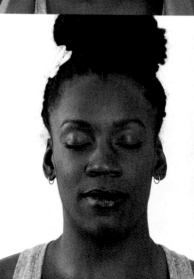

5

With your thumbs and the side of your index fingers closest to your thumbs, gently pinch your ears—start at your earlobes, move up to the top and back down to your earlobes a couple times.

6

End by fluttering your lips as you exhale.

RELAX YOUR BACK

Child's Pose

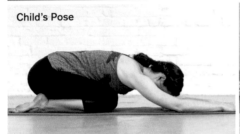

Supported Twist

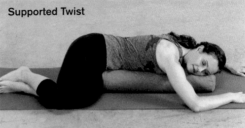

Relaxation Pose

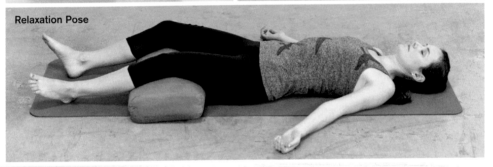

Reclined Hero

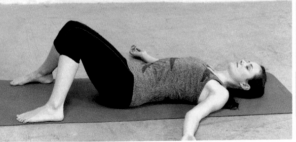

Constructive Rest

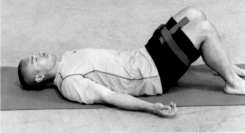

Restorative Bridge

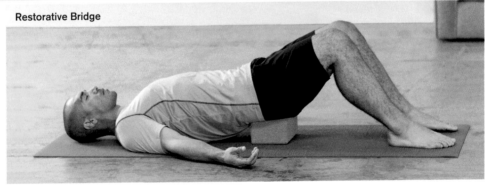

LENGTHEN YOUR BODY

Surfer

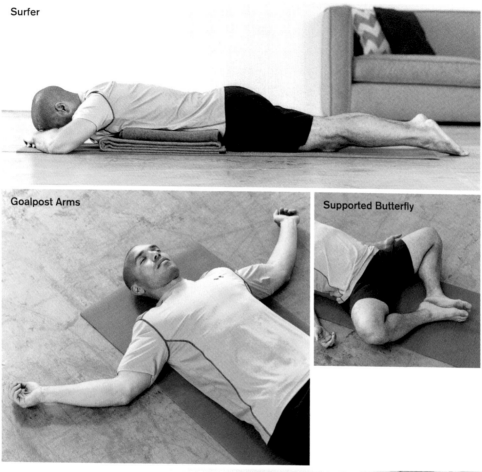

Goalpost Arms

Supported Butterfly

Supported Bridge

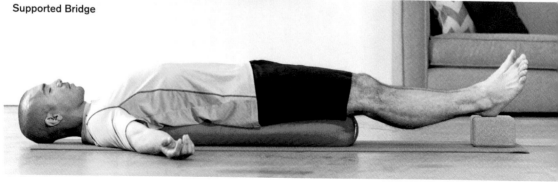

FULL BODY MOBILITY

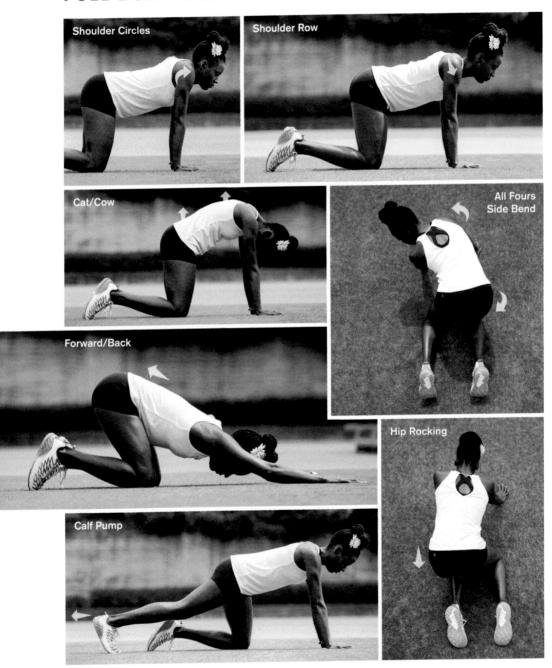

Shoulder Circles

Shoulder Row

Cat/Cow

All Fours Side Bend

Forward/Back

Hip Rocking

Calf Pump

RECOVERY BOOST

Butterfly at the Wall

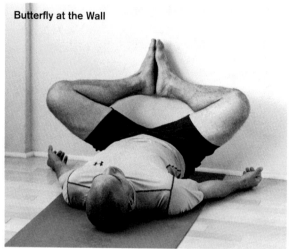

Figure 4 at the Wall

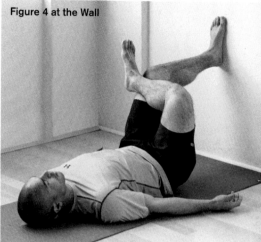

Legs Up the Wall

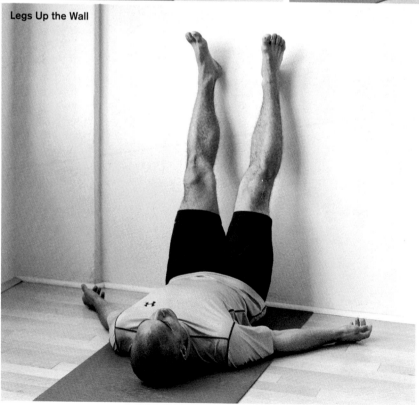

Coping with Injury

For athletes—and everyone—injury is inevitable. And it sucks. But it doesn't have to be devastating. Consider the fact that what might seem like a major setback could instead be an important opportunity to pause, take stock of where you're at, and adjust your plans accordingly.

We're usually going so hard in the pursuit of our goals that it can be easy to lose track of what our body is telling us. We move so fast we blow right past sensations—aches, pains, niggles—that are our body's requests to pay closer attention and respond accordingly. Or we're so fixated on the goal itself, we choose to ignore these important cues because we're scared they will derail our plans.

It can be hard psychologically to acknowledge red flags and, ultimately, injuries themselves. But there is nothing to fear. Your body is incredibly resilient, and bringing a positive attitude to your rehab will greatly aid the healing process.

Rather than panicking about your injury, consider approaching it as an invitation back to balance—an opportunity to pause and address what ails you, knowing that ultimately you will be stronger for it. A positive, receptive mental state will optimize your healing. Injuries ask us to work in.

Approach injury as an invitation *back to balance.*

GET REAL

If you are injured, ask yourself:

How can I be more receptive to what my body or this injury is telling me?

How can I work in to optimize the healing process?

How can I grow from this injury?

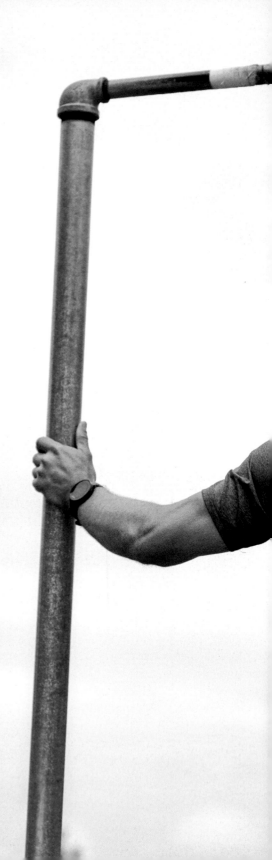

04

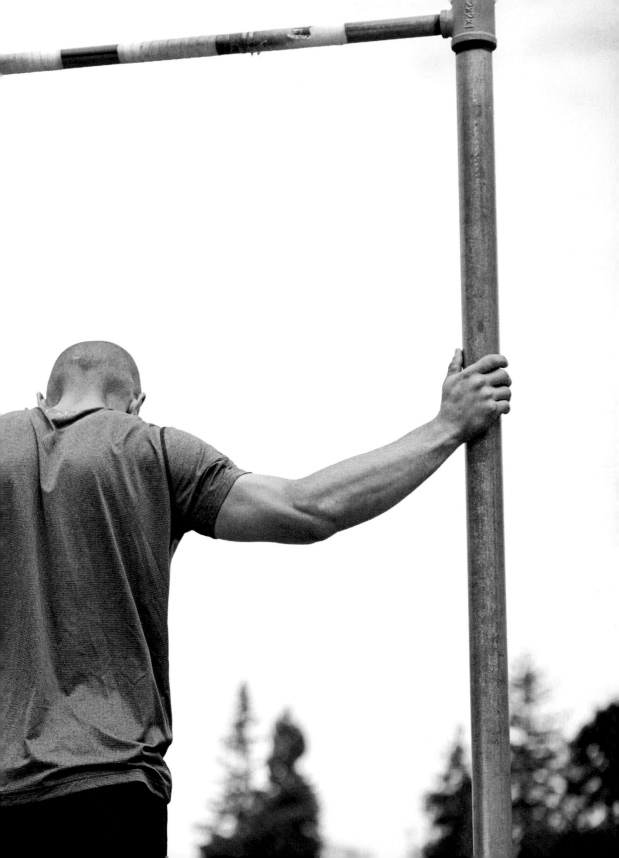

THE PLAN: RECOVER FOR REAL

More than anything, "the plan" is to just start—start making recovery a priority and get real about how to make it happen. Or, perhaps more accurately, just stop—stop talking about how tired you are and do something about it. The more seamlessly you can integrate recovery into your real, everyday life—in the moments when you need it most—the better you will feel and the more energy you will have while you work hard . . . and the more effective you will be in everything you do. That's what real recovery is all about.

The goal of this 4-week, 28-day plan is to help you put the meditation and restorative yoga tools in this book to use in a meaningful way. It's designed to help you establish a consistent practice of mental focus and physical relaxation and, ultimately, develop an intentional, realistic approach to recovery.

Each week includes:
⇒ A clear restorative focus to make your recovery sessions more purposeful
⇒ A tangible mental focus tool to build practical meditation skills
⇒ Related meditation routines to become familiar with and practice different techniques
⇒ Accompanying restorative yoga postures to recharge your body and maximize the benefits of your sessions

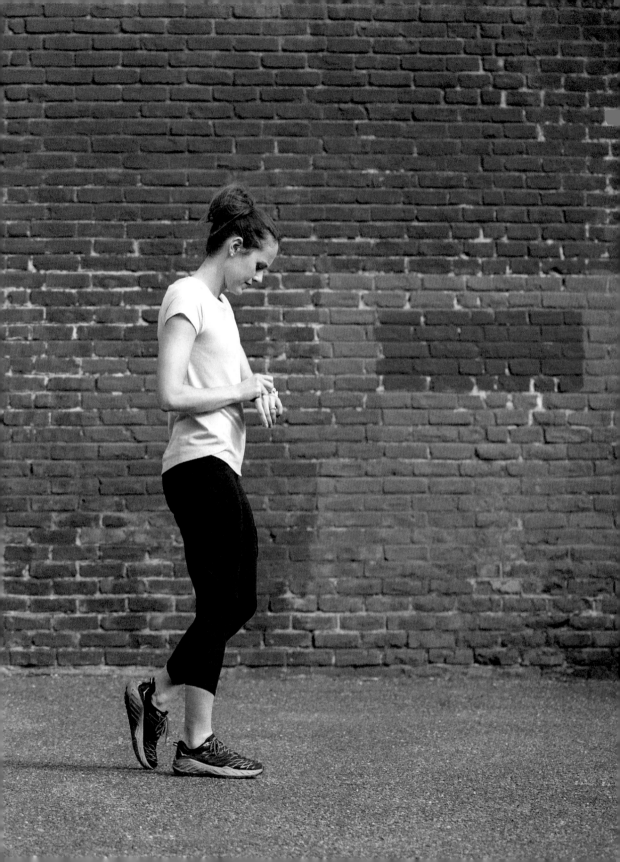

This chapter includes additional prompts to help you make recovery work for you, and it has space to note your intentions and observations if you feel inspired, which will help you further ground what you're doing and, more important, see why. It's this understanding that ultimately sparks motivation for continual practice.

Each day, this plan recommends a meditation with an accompanying yoga posture. While you shouldn't approach recovery rigidly, do commit to completing the entire month of pairings to give yourself the opportunity to learn and practice these key restorative tools and set yourself up for success moving forward.

Then, use the provided tips and inspiration to transition from this starter plan to make your own plan—using these tools to work in and recover for real.

Are you ready to work in?

Your athletic potential is waiting for you to say yes.

GET REAL

My goal for the month ahead is:

I'm using this plan because:

I'll stay on track over the next month by:

COMMIT

Your focus this week is to commit to recovery. Make the commitment to yourself, and honor it over the course of the month—make it a non-negotiable priority. It doesn't matter if you spend 2 minutes or 20, or 2 hours; the most important thing is that you commit to make recovery happen every day. This week, set aside whatever time you can, wherever it fits into your day. This could vary from day to day, which is fine.

TOOL

Breathe (pp. 31–32)

MEDITATION

Use breath-focused meditations to become aware of how your breathing supports recovery.

⇒ Awareness Breath (p. 48)

⇒ Humming Breath (p. 54)

⇒ Belly Breath (p. 52)

⇒ Extended Exhalation Breath (p. 50)

YOGA

Open the front of your body to become more receptive to restorative practice.

⇒ Goalpost Arms (p. 104)

⇒ Relaxation Pose (p. 106)

⇒ Supported Butterfly (p. 114)

⇒ Restorative Bridge (p. 108)

	Whenever it fits into your day, set a timer for the duration of time you have available/want to spend.
HOW TO DO IT	⇒ Pause and notice how you feel.
	⇒ Do the meditation and restorative yoga in unison.
	⇒ Pause and notice how you feel.

DAILY PLAN

DAY	DAY	DAY	DAY
Awareness Breath + Goalpost Arms	Humming Breath + Relaxation Pose	Belly Breath + Supported Butterfly	Humming Breath + Relaxation Pose

DAY	DAY	DAY
Belly Breath + Supported Butterfly	Extended Exhalation Breath ⟵ + Restorative Bridge ⟶	

Match your desire to achieve your goals

with your *commitment to working in.*

GET REAL

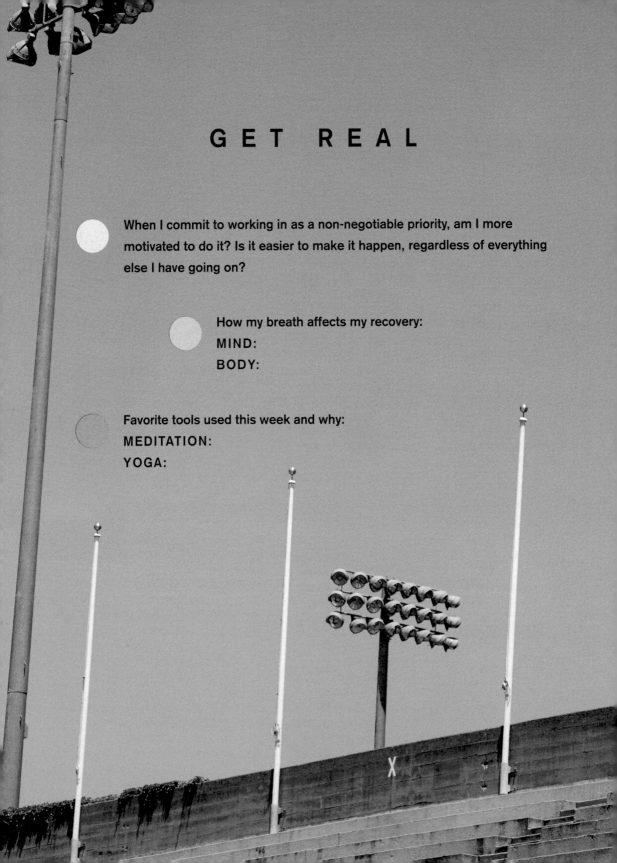

When I commit to working in as a non-negotiable priority, am I more motivated to do it? Is it easier to make it happen, regardless of everything else I have going on?

How my breath affects my recovery:
MIND:
BODY:

Favorite tools used this week and why:
MEDITATION:
YOGA:

BE CONSISTENT

This week create consistency in the way in which you work in. Like anything, recovery takes consistent practice for it to pay off. In addition, creating consistency in your approach can make a big difference in terms of both finding a way to fit it in and making it effective. Last week you worked in whenever it best fit in—which was likely not the same time every day. This week set aside the same amount of time at the same time daily to help build the habit and solidify it as part of your routine. Obviously, there will be times when you need to flex it (managing this reality is next week's focus), but this week, focus your restorative time and energy in a consistent manner.

⇒ **Begin by selecting your restorative mantra for the week (flip back to pp. 56–61 for inspiration)**

TOOL	Speak (p. 32)
MEDITATION	Strengthen your restorative intention and resolve. ⇒ **Mantra Meditation (p. 56)**
YOGA	Become familiar with "the boss" of restorative yoga, knowing that this is the best pose to default to. ⇒ **Legs Up the Wall (p. 128)**

Continues

<table>
<tr><td>

HOW TO DO IT

</td><td>

At the same time every day, set a timer for the duration of time you will spend. Spend the same amount of time on each session.

⇒ Pause and notice how you feel.

⇒ Put your Legs Up the Wall and do the Mantra Meditation, incorporating your restorative mantra.

⇒ Pause and notice how you feel.

</td></tr>
</table>

DAILY PLAN	DAY 8	DAY 9	DAY 10	DAY 11
	⟵————— Mantra Meditation + Legs Up the Wall —————⟶			

DAY 12	DAY 13	DAY 14
⟵——— Mantra Meditation + Legs Up the Wall ———⟶		

Be consistent in your input.

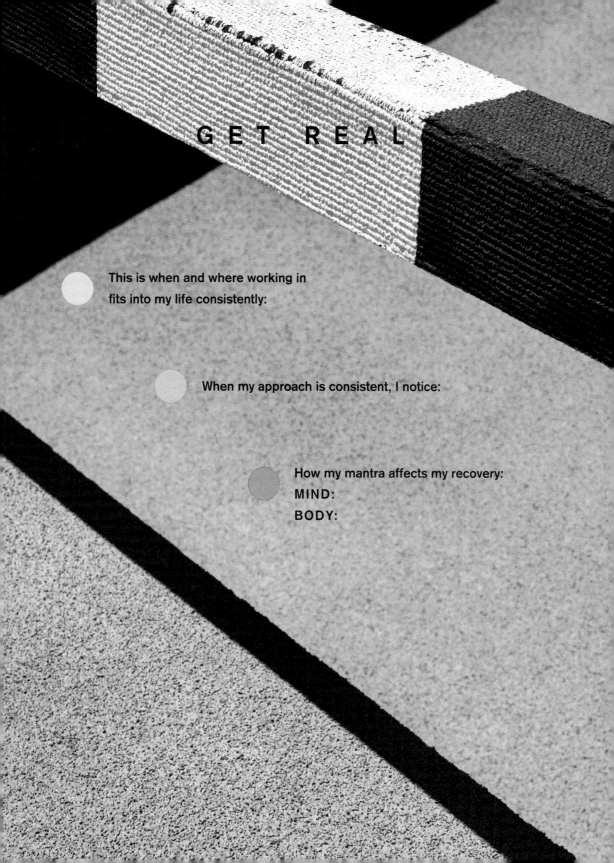

GET REAL

This is when and where working in
fits into my life consistently:

When my approach is consistent, I notice:

How my mantra affects my recovery:
MIND:
BODY:

MEET THE CHALLENGE

By this week your motivation might start to wane, or maybe something unexpected has happened in your schedule or training. This is your chance to meet any challenge you perceive more easefully, strengthen your mind, and become more resilient in the process.

TOOL

See (p. 32)

MEDITATION

Use visualization to sharpen your mental focus and overcome obstacles.

⇒ **Let Go Visualization (p. 62)**

⇒ **Recovery Visualization (p. 64)**

⇒ **Taper Visualization (p. 66)**

YOGA

Support yourself with key restorative poses that hold you up and create more space in your body to meet and transcend the unfamiliarity and potential accompanying discomfort of deep physical relaxation.

⇒ **Surfer (p. 120)**

⇒ **Supported Child's Pose (p. 98)**

⇒ **Supported Forward Fold (p. 118)**

HOW TO DO IT	Whenever it fits into your day, set a timer for the duration of time you have available or how much time you want to spend.

⇒ **Pause and notice how you feel in the context of any challenges you are managing.**

⇒ **Do the meditation and restorative yoga in unison.**

⇒ **Pause and notice how you feel—specifically notice your outlook about your challenge.**

DAILY PLAN

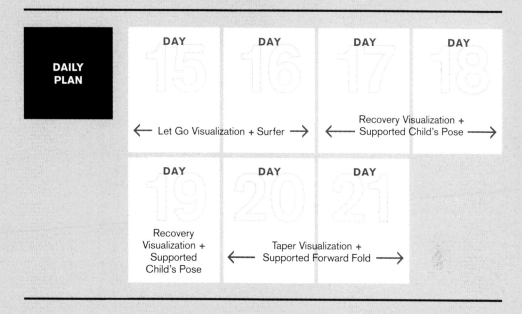

DAY 15	DAY 16	DAY 17	DAY 18
← Let Go Visualization + Surfer →		Recovery Visualization + Supported Child's Pose →	

DAY 19	DAY 20	DAY 21
Recovery Visualization + Supported Child's Pose	← Taper Visualization + Supported Forward Fold →	

Work in to manage any challenge

more easefully.

GET REAL

When I work in, this is what I notice about my ability to manage challenges:

How my sight/visualization affects my recovery:

MIND:

BODY:

Favorite tools used this week and why:

MEDITATION:

YOGA:

This week feel the sensations of recovery and the accompanying ease. Embrace them and be them as your sessions become more effective. The more spacious and restful you feel, the more you are in fact recovering. You will use your felt sense in meditation and restorative yoga that gently mobilizes to create a more tangible, tactile quality to your practice.

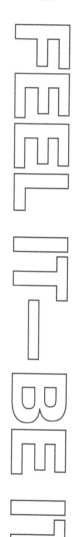

TOOL	Feel (p. 32)

MEDITATION	Use your felt sense in meditation to help you decrease tension and explore physical sensations that support optimal recovery.

⇒ Dissolve Tension Meditation (p. 70)

⇒ Feeling Meditation (p. 68)

⇒ Cooling Meditation (p. 74)

⇒ Create Space Meditation (p. 72)

Continues

YOGA

Increase fluidity in muscles, surrounding tissues, and joints to help ease stiffness and restore range of motion as you relax your body.

⇒ Shoulder Circles (p. 134)

⇒ Neck Circles (p. 130)

⇒ Shoulder Row (p. 138)

⇒ Cat/Cow (p. 140)

⇒ All Fours Side Bend (p. 142)

⇒ Windshield Wipers (p. 150)

⇒ Forward/Back (p. 144)

⇒ Hip Rocking (p. 146)

HOW TO DO IT

Whenever it fits into your day, set a timer for the duration of time you have available or how much time you want to spend.

⇒ Pause and notice how you feel.

⇒ Do the restorative yoga and then do the meditation during the remaining time.

⇒ Pause and notice how you feel.

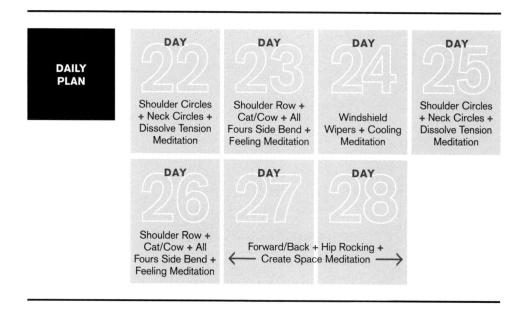

DAILY PLAN

DAY 22
Shoulder Circles + Neck Circles + Dissolve Tension Meditation

DAY 23
Shoulder Row + Cat/Cow + All Fours Side Bend + Feeling Meditation

DAY 24
Windshield Wipers + Cooling Meditation

DAY 25
Shoulder Circles + Neck Circles + Dissolve Tension Meditation

DAY 26
Shoulder Row + Cat/Cow + All Fours Side Bend + Feeling Meditation

DAY 27 / DAY 28
← Forward/Back + Hip Rocking + Create Space Meditation →

If you can *feel it*, you can *be it.*

GET REAL

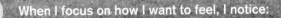

When I focus on how I want to feel, I notice:

How my felt sense affects my recovery:
MIND:
BODY:

Favorite tools used this week and why:
MEDITATION:
YOGA:

When I'm busy and can't be bothered to devote time and attention to recovery, I will default to _____ to make it happen.

One thing I can do anytime, anywhere—right now— to recharge is:

How will I be more aware of when I need to stop?

When I do stop, how will I recover for real?

Keep Going: The Real Plan

Hopefully by this point you've become more aware of your current recovery habits or lack thereof—that's a big step in the right direction.

As you complete this month-long plan, continue to absorb your restorative input and resolve to continue. Now is the time to begin your own practice—keep it practical for your life so that you're empowered to make it happen, regardless of what path you're on or where you hope it will lead. Be fluid in your approach, knowing that anything is better than nothing and that your consistent input—a little bit every day—is what will refuel you for your best possible output.

The plan from here is to keep working in so that you can keep working out. Approach the two not as "training and not training" but as equally important and productive aspects of effort that work best as a unit to move you toward your goals. The more you can master working in, the greater command you will have over all your systems and the more effective your recovery will be.

Use the worksheets on the following pages as needed for further inspiration and grounding as you continue to work in and optimize everything you do.

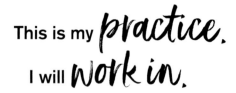

This is my *practice.*
I will *work in.*

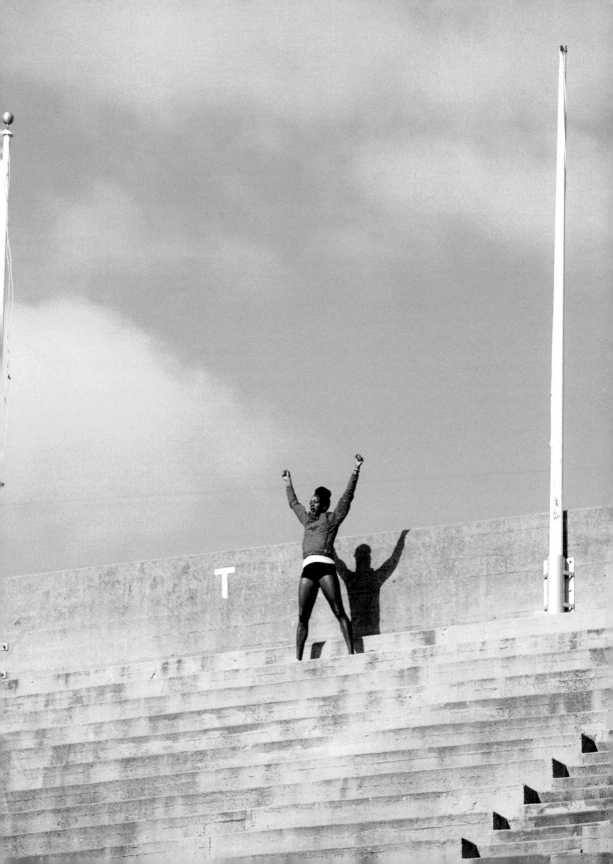

WORK IN

FOCUS

Intentional mental transition—daily meditation to shift from training to recovering

Support body during high-mileage week—daily legs up restorative yoga poses to promote recovery

DAILY PLAN

MON.	**TUES.**	**WED.**
Mantra Meditation + Legs Up the Couch	Belly Breath + Supported Bridge	Mantra Meditation + Legs Up the Couch

THURS.	**FRI.**	**SAT.**	**SUN.**
Belly Breath + Supported Bridge	Create Space Meditation + Legs Up the Wall	Let Go Visualization + Recovery Boost Routine	Recovery Visualization + Recovery Boost Routine

GET REAL

Just like I don't always feel like working out, I don't always feel like working in. But I usually feel satisfied and proud of myself when I push through and work out anyway, and I'm getting similar results from working in.

It's worth the effort, and I keep reminding myself that so I get it done.

The more I recover for real, the more my body demands it, especially during high-mileage weeks. And the more I practice, the more efficient I'm becoming at making the transition from work to rest. I'm getting better every time I work in and it feels great.

WEEK ____

WORK IN

FOCUS

DAILY PLAN

MON.	TUES.	WED.

THURS.	FRI.	SAT.	SUN.

GET REAL

WEEK
_____

WORK IN

FOCUS

DAILY PLAN

MON.	TUES.	WED.

THURS.	FRI.	SAT.	SUN.

GET REAL

WORK IN

FOCUS

DAILY PLAN

| MON. | TUES. | WED. |

| THURS. | FRI. | SAT. | SUN. |

GET REAL

WEEK
____

WORK IN

FOCUS

DAILY PLAN

MON.

TUES.

WED.

THURS.

FRI.

SAT.

SUN.

GET REAL

WEEK

WORK IN

FOCUS

DAILY PLAN

| MON. | TUES. | WED. |

| THURS. | FRI. | SAT. | SUN. |

GET REAL

HIGH FIVES

I wrote this book because I felt called to help athletes create a real plan to recover more efficiently and effectively from the demands of sport and life. I've long believed in our innate ability to push hard, accomplish more, and realize our dreams not by gritting our teeth and grinding harder, but by taking a deeper breath and creating space to recharge even as we work. Early in the process of writing **WORK IN**, I put this mantra on the wall:

Relax as I work

Nothing has affirmed this belief for me more than this project. Over the course of the last year, during which I've held myself accountable to these practices, I have become more easeful and steady, and as a result more energized and productive than ever before. I found that writing this book felt like medicine—both preventative and regenerative.

There are many people without whose support this project would not have been possible and who help me in so many ways to serve my mission of helping as many athletes as possible use yoga to achieve their goals. Publishing a book is a team effort and I'm so thankful for my squad.

Thank you to my husband and north star Mark Taylor for your love, support, vision, and dot connecting. Thank you to my daughter Rose who, more than anyone else, has underscored for me the importance of working in. I created this book in a year of her naptimes and, thankfully, she slept like a champ.

Thank you to all my teachers, with special gratitude to Richelle Ricard for being my anatomy guru, Elena Brower for being a lighthouse, Jane Fryer for trailblazing, Susie Johns for keeping it real, and Hanya Chlala for helping me stay balanced.

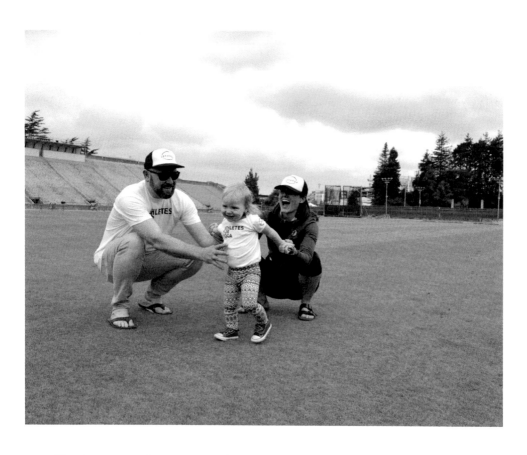

Thank you to photographer Claire Pepper for capturing the magic, colleague Sarah "Mac" Robinson for having my back, my editor Renee Jardine and her VeloPress crew for guidance and belief, and the women of Oiselle for empowerment, plus the flyest styles around.

Like all of my content, **WORK IN** would not be what it is without the athletes. To Alysia Montaño, thank you for your leadership. I have so much gratitude and respect for Alysia and Louis Montaño for leading us through the pages of this book.

And most importantly, thank you for being an Athlete for Yoga. High fives for picking up this book. Know that you are leading by example and helping many others every time you take a deep breath in . . . and a slow breath out. . . .

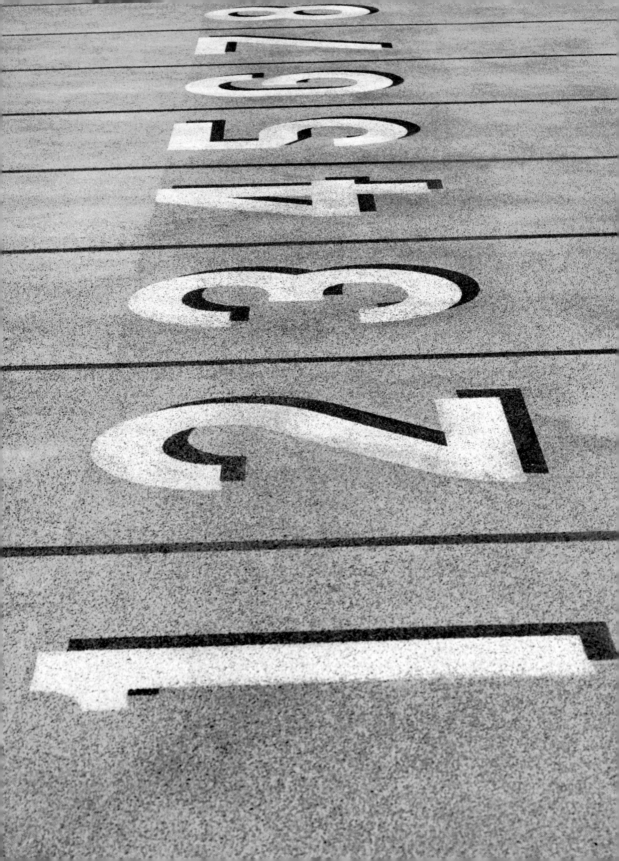

ABOUT THE ATHLETES

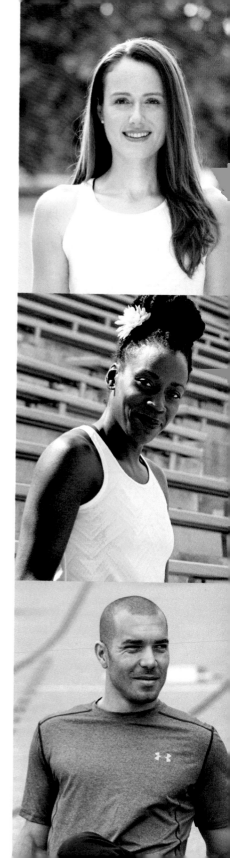

ERIN TAYLOR

A former collegiate basketball player, Erin helps athletes use yoga to achieve their goals. As a new mom, she gets her workout stroller running, and she doesn't mind sharing her yoga mat with her toddler. She believes that when it comes to yoga, the more real the yoga, the bigger the impact.

ALYSIA MONTAÑO

A 2012 Olympian, Alysia is a seven-time USA champion in the 800 meters who wears a flower in her hair to signify strength. Her philosophy in sport and life is to be bold and courageous, and she's known for uplifting and inspiring athletes of all kinds. She also loves a Legs Up the Wall session.

LOUIS MONTAÑO

Fitness instructor, filmmaker, and partner to Alysia, Lou is always working on his fitness and finding ways to find balance in sport, family, and life. When it comes to working in, he's a pro.

ABOUT THE AUTHOR

Erin Taylor is an international leader in yoga for athletes. Her mission is to help as many athletes as possible use yoga to achieve their goals, and become more balanced and resilient along the way.

It was her own experience of being sidelined by injury as a collegiate basketball player that first showed her how yoga can be the reset that brings athletes back into balance. Erin founded Jasyoga to equip athletes with powerful skills to prevent injuries and enhance recovery, optimizing performance in sport and life. Over the last decade, she has infused meditation, functional anatomy, and physical therapy techniques into her practice. Now accessible anytime, anywhere via her online video platform and her book **HIT RESET**, Erin's approach has been widely embraced by athletes ranging from recreational to elite, and can be configured to help anyone achieve their goals.

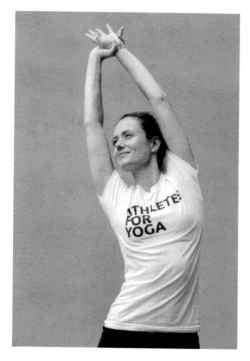

In addition to privately coaching sports teams and athletes, she hosts yoga-for-athletes certification programs and writes a popular blog at jasyoga.com/blog. She lives in London with her husband and daughter.